The *girlfriends* DIET

The *girlfriends* DIET

Burn More Calories on a Delicious 4-Week Mediterranean Meal Plan

FROM THE EDITORS OF GOOD HOUSEKEEPING

Hearst Editions
New York

Contents

PART 1

The Girlfriends Way to Diet & Live

PART 2

The Girlfriends Meal Plan & Recipes

Foreword

HERE'S THE THING ABOUT MOST DIETS: They're kind of a drag. You pledge to eat less, move more, and after a few weeks of denying yourself the happiness that is a sleeve of candy-colored macaroons and devoting yourself to the elliptical machine, maybe, just maybe, you drop a couple of pounds. Then what? If you're truly self-motivated, you keep up the good work. The rest of us (me!) revert to bad habits. But you can change this pattern with the help of GH's proven new weight-loss plan. I did! And the make-it-stick trick is simple: Enlist the support of a girlfriend(s). Research proves that dieters who team up to slim down are more likely to lose weight for good. Why? Well, there's the accountability factor. Are you really going to blow off Zumba when you know your friend is there waiting for you? No. Plus, it's more fun. Yes, I did say, fun. Because The Girlfriends Diet is just that and that's why it works. Throughout this book, you'll be inspired by real women's stories of remarkable body transformations. You'll learn their secrets and be given the tools to rev your own metabolism, burn more calories and eat smarter without ever feeling deprived. (You might want to skip directly to page 293 for the Chocolate Pudding Cake recipe. Just saying.) So, whether you have 5, 15, 25 pounds or more to lose, grab a friend and let the slim begin right here, right now…with a smile.

Jane

Jane Francisco
Editor in Chief, *Good Housekeeping*

PART 1

The Girlfriends Way to Diet & Live

Meet Your New Best Friends

CHRISTI BORCHERS was lumbering through her 30s at 200-and-something pounds until a chance run-in with an old friend ended in a pact that they'd both get fit together. Today, Christi not only is 80 pounds lighter, but you can find her at the head of the Zumba class that she once hid in the back of—now as the instructor. (Find the rest of Christi's story on page 172.)

Give it up for Jackie Freitag, who got the much-needed kick in her size 20 pants when her close friend asked her to be her maid of honor. "It was like, ugh, I can't be the fat girl of the wedding party," she remembers oh so well. Not only did her BFF, her fiancé, and her gal pals at her old gym support her journey to a 105-pound weight loss, but they were cheering her on when she finished running two marathons. (Read more about Jackie on page 44.)

Another cheer goes to Vicki Baughman, who couldn't figure out any way to get out of her size 28 clothes until she started getting on a treadmill and sharing diet secrets and advice with a group of virtual girlfriends. Today, they are all marveling over her photos in her now size 2 pencil skirts. (There's more about Vicki on page 26.)

You may never actually meet any of these extraordinary women in person, but you'll get to feel as though you know them as you read their compelling and triumphant stories in the coming pages. They, and dozens of other women like them who first shared their dieting successes and secrets in the pages of magazines like *Good Housekeeping*, *Redbook*, *Marie Claire*, *Cosmopolitan* and *Woman's Day*, are appearing once again in these pages to inspire you with their stories and successful dieting tips so you, too, can make your weight-loss dream come true. Consider them your diet buddies— your new best friends who will inspire you to steadily and assuredly lose a pound or more a week until you reach the weight you want, just as they did. It doesn't matter if you're trying to lose 10, 20, 50 or 100 pounds; as you'll learn, your chances of weight-loss success increase dramatically when you diet with friends.

Diet Teams Work Best

Though from disparate backgrounds and different parts of the country, these women all share a common bond. They finally and permanently took off the weight they struggled for decades to lose by realizing what it actually takes to get there: a commitment to a new lifestyle of healthy eating, regular daily activity and a support group that is with you all the way. They'll all tell you that the key to ditching their old habits in favor of healthy ones was the motivation they got from their supporters—be it spouse, kids, coworkers, friends, diet buddies or online cheerleaders. It's the same kind of discovery, friendship and bonding that can help you, too.

Talk to any woman who's ever tried to break a bad habit, and she'll tell you the process can be tough *and* isolating. However, what these women have discovered, research proves: Support is the key to success—and that's especially true when it comes to weight loss.

According to the American Psychological Association, your chances of losing weight and keeping it off are best when you have a social network where you can share tips on diet and exercise *and* when you have a diet buddy or buddies to go along with you for the ride, just as you will on The Girlfriends Diet. Brown University researchers found that people who had a diet buddy dropped significantly more weight after a year of effort compared with those who went it alone. When people are in a group with others on the same journey and make themselves accountable to one another, they feel there is this element of, *Hey, this worked for her, so why can't it work for me, too? I'm giving it a try!*

While getting support and diet directives (eat this, don't eat that) from a professional—be it your doctor or a well-established forum such as Weight Watchers—beats doing it on your own, dieter-helping-dieter has proved to produce the best results. In another study at Brown University Medical School, meeting with a health coach helped dieters shed almost 10% of their weight in six months. But, the researchers discovered, the counselor didn't have to be anyone official: A diet buddy—a so-called peer coach—worked just as well.

A diet buddy can be even more effective than a professional. University of Pittsburgh researchers put this theory to the test by pitting dieting teams of four friends against lone dieters, all of whom were given the same eating plan and the same behavioral counseling. Among the loners, 76% completed the program and 24% went on to maintain their weight loss after 10 months. But 95% of the diet buddies completed the program, and 66% maintained their full weight loss 10 months later, way overshooting the 20% long-term success rate that is believed to be the norm. A lot of it has to do with accountability, research shows. Being in it together gives you a feeling of responsibility to others—you don't want to let them down. And it appears to work best peer to peer.

Another study involving more than 200 people, most of whom were women, found that professionally led diet programs can actually hinder weight-loss progress because they tend to be so rigid. However, even in such a setting, the dropout rate is lower when friends attend the program together. More important, the researchers discovered the same thing: Friends dieting together manage to keep the weight off longer than individuals who make a go of it alone. In the study group, two-thirds of diet buddies were still successful six months later, compared with only a quarter of those who were on their own. Long lasting, just like a friendship.

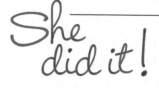

RITA COOKSON
AGE **42**
LOST **29 POUNDS!**

HERE'S HOW: "I look at wedding pictures and think, *Oh! Is that me?* My mother has said, 'Well, what do you expect? You're a mom and a wife now. You're never going to look like that again.' I don't think that has to be the case. I'm a pastry chef, and I come from a big Italian family that loves to eat, so making a healthier diet a part of my lifestyle is always going to be key. It was that nudge from my mom that set my mind to doing it.

"If I can lose weight, anyone can! Last year at this time, I felt depressed, tired and generally gross about myself. I am a completely different person today. I stopped eating all those extra cupcakes and cookies, plus I have my exercise buddies. I've been doing four fun cardio classes per week, in addition to meeting with a trainer twice a week.

"I was afraid of lifting heavy weights because I thought I'd bulk up, but I got leaner and feel amazing. My husband climbed the Canadian Rockies last summer, but I didn't go because I wasn't in that kind of shape. Now, maybe I can go with him!"

Man, Woman, Food, Diet

Girlfriends share a special closeness that is quite different from male bonding. Studies show there is a direct relationship between emotional support and psychological well-being—something that benefits both genders. However, while male and female friendship networks are similar with regard to quality and trust, studies show that women benefit much more from their relationships with other women in terms of their health pursuits, especially when it comes to weight loss, simply because they are much more willing to make the effort to go on a diet and eat better.

One reason relates to the different ways we perceive our bodies. "Women are more dissatisfied with their body weight and shape than men," says Barbara J. Rolls, Ph.D., an expert in food and gender differences and professor at Pennsylvania State University. In one Florida study, when both sexes were asked to critique their own bodies, the men thought they'd be "too skinny" at the weight the health charts said they should be and just shrugged it off. Women who were at their ideal weight, according to the charts, thought they weren't skinny enough and that men would like to see them even thinner than they were. The guys didn't agree with the women's view of themselves.

Women simply have their minds on their weight a lot more than men, according to a study published in the *British Food Journal*. A lot of men only start getting antsy about their weight and decide they better do something about it when they are hit with a health threat—like a heart attack scare, or high cholesterol or blood pressure. Same goes for women, too, but they are just as likely to want to lose weight in response to a threat to their psychological well-being—like a skinny frenemy who appears to be having more fun. It's just the way a lot of us are wired.

Women tend to benefit more from weight-loss support groups

because, in general, our gender is more susceptible to the unrealistic messages magazines, television and Hollywood send out about what is "acceptable" thinness and beauty. Support networks can help keep us in touch with reality—a key component to success because unrealistic weight-loss expectations are a driver of weight-loss failure.

Then there are the differences in our relationship with food. In general, men go for meat and potatoes, and women like carbs—salads, pasta and sweets. Comfort food? Men want steaks, casseroles and chili, while women think of comfort as chocolate and ice cream. In food survey questionnaires, women report they like and eat fruits, vegetables and fish, but when we're under stress and the going gets rocky, these are the foods we give up—and we break out the cookies. In fact, one study reported in *Health Psychology* found that when men get stressed out, they "markedly and significantly" get turned off by food, but women eat nearly *twice* as much. *Yikes!*

Guys, in general, have a hard time understanding the relationship women have with food. We are more motivated to eat healthy foods and much more determined when we set out to lose weight—which experts say explains 50% of gender differences in food choices. "Women experience more food-related conflict than men in that they like fattening foods but perceive that they should not eat them," says Rolls. When we cave in, it sends us on a guilt trip. Men just dive in and enjoy.

This is not to say that guys and gals can't be diet buddies. Or that a man can't be your chief supporter. Many of the women in this book are proof of that. Spouses are important to weight-loss success—and it works both ways. But if you pair up with a guy, you have to realize that, when it comes to dieting, men and women are not on an equal playing field. It doesn't necessarily come any easier to men, but they do lose weight faster. Meaning it can be hard not to start resenting your significant other when he eats foot-long subs and still drops five pounds, while you nibble on nothing but salads and lose only one. There's a biological reason for this: When it comes to metabolism, men have it made.

"Men naturally have more lean muscle, so their metabolic rates run about 10% faster than women's," says Liz Applegate, Ph.D., director of sports nutrition at the University of California, Davis. "Women's bodies, on the other hand, are designed to hold on to body fat to nurture and grow babies."

Men's body composition is another reason they have the easier-losing edge. Men have more muscle mass and about 10% less body fat than women. Muscle burns at least twice as many calories as fat, even when you're just sitting around doing nothing. In fact, one study found that men naturally burn 37% more calories per day

High-Protein Diets Are Not Female-Friendly

Ever try a high-protein, low-carbohydrate diet? How long did it last for you? A week? Two? Even less?

There's a reason why women cannot tolerate a high-protein, low-carb diet very well, says Olga Raz, M.Sc., R.D., a diet researcher from Israel and author of *The Bread for Life Diet*. And it all has to do with our biology.

Compared with men, women naturally have lower levels of serotonin, the hormone that controls satiety. Eating carbs is what gives our serotonin a lift. "When serotonin levels are low, we get cravings and feel hungry," says Raz. In her research she's found that robbing ourselves of carbohydrates—the good kind found in foods like vegetables and whole grains—makes serotonin levels sink even lower. "I have women patients who tell me they can't tolerate a low-carb diet like Atkins, but their husbands do not have a problem sticking with it," she says. On the other hand, a diet high in complex carbs, like you'll find on The Girlfriends Diet, raises serotonin levels, so you'll feel fuller longer.

through movement than women. Plus, there's some evidence that female hormones, estrogen in particular, encourage our bodies to store food as fat, especially around the middle.

The bottom line? You can diet with your significant other or best guy pal to keep each other encouraged and motivated, just don't go in a head-to-head competition with each other. But if you're in need of help from someone who can truly connect with what you're going through—biologically and mentally—some girl-to-girl bonding is to your benefit. And there's a place to find it even if your BFF is a "perfect" size 6.

Dieter Meet Dieter

Emerging research shows that social networking your way to weight loss works. In one study conducted by The George Washington University School of Nursing, 349 Oregon workers joined a company-run website with the goal to improve health-related behavior. After six months, the online users increased the time they spent walking by 164%, compared with only 47% in another group of workers who tried the same endeavor offline. And though the goal was to improve overall healthfulness and not to lose weight per se, the online users lost an average of 5.2 pounds, compared with an average of only 1.5 pounds in the offline folks.

Another study, conducted by Baylor College of Medicine, found that dieters who were given access to three diet tools—group meetings, a mobile app and online services—lost nearly eight times more weight (10.1 pounds versus just 1.3 pounds) after six months than people who tried to diet on their own.

Group weight loss is so powerful that even videoconferencing works. In one three-month experiment that took place in South Dakota, people who met and supported each other once a week with a videoconference meeting lost weight, while another group that went on the same diet on their own *gained* weight.

Other studies have also found that mobile apps and instant messaging are valuable, especially when it comes to maintaining weight loss. In one study, Duke University researchers sent out a daily 8 A.M. message to 120 successful dieters who had already lost an average of 15 pounds. Three months later, *everyone* had still maintained their new weight. It's a reinforcement technique, the researchers concluded, that shows promise in helping people "sustain healthy behaviors that can lead to improved health outcomes."

ADVICE FROM A BESTIE

Keep your 'before' pictures."

"When you're losing weight, your day-to-day progress can be slow, and it's easy to think nothing's happening. So I tell my friends, don't ditch the fat photos! When you look at a picture of your former self, it's a lot easier to see what transformation has taken place. On days when I feel like blowing off the gym, my 'before' pics remind me of how hard I've worked and that I didn't get here by making excuses or giving in to temptation. That makes me stronger."

—*Antoinette Marrero, 33, Metuchen, NJ, who lost 45 pounds*

The same opportunities can be yours when you team up with a friend or group of friends and go on The Girlfriends Diet and form your own Girlfriends Diet Club, a female-focused approach to healthy weight loss that combines a Mediterranean-style eating plan, behavior-modification strategies and exercise. You'll team up together in a mutual effort to:

* Increase your intake of fruits, vegetables, legumes and whole grains

"I post my weekly progress on Facebook. My girlfriends' 'likes' encourage me to carry on."
— *Wendy Kalman, facebook.com/goodhousekeeping*

Calling All Girlfriends

You can meet virtual like-minded dieters by connecting with any number of online diet groups and bloggers. You can do it alone and join an established group of like-minded dieters, or you can form your own Girlfriends Diet Club to work as a team online.

It's a strategy many studies reveal can lead to success. Michelle and Brian Coleman, 42-year-old marrieds and diet buddies, decided to form a social media diet support group on Facebook after the pair lost a combined amazing 254 pounds. "We launched with five friends, and it's grown to 35 members," Michelle reports. "We motivate one another and share ideas about how to overcome obstacles. Several people have lost more than 10% of their body weight—and one member was so inspired that she signed up for her first triathlon."

These are a few of the other websites women featured in this book recommend:

Sparkpeople.com—With more than 13 million members, this may just be the largest collection of successful losers in the world. Even with so many people, it's still fairly easy to find and work with others who match your goals.

Weightlossbuddy.com—Connect, inspire and lose weight together. It's all here. You might even become the weight-loss buddy of the month.

Meetup.com—Type in keywords like "weight loss" or "walking," and connect with a support group that meets face-to-face. Can't find a fit? Choose the "Start a Meetup Group" tab to launch a new one in your area.

Myfitnesspal.com—Sign up for a free membership, and you'll gain access to discussion forums where you can find support from others who are in the process of making healthy lifestyle changes. Bonus: The site also gives you an online food diary, a searchable food database and free mobile apps to keep track of your exercise and calorie intake on the go.

Exercisefriends.com—Enter your zip code, age and the type of activity you're interested in, and you'll be connected with potential exercise buddies. Then you can set a date for an in-person meeting.

* Incorporate more activity into your daily life, including walking and other easy forms of exercise

* Break bad habits around food

* Deal with stress in ways that will not drive you to food

* Take more time for yourself to improve your health and well-being

* Use girlfriend power for support to keep you motivated and on track

Think of the weight-loss potential: A lot to lose and nothing to gain! The blueprint to get you started—the diet, recipes and exercise plan—is the book you have in your hands right now.

Starting a Club of Your Own

Starting a Girlfriends Diet Club is simple. All you need is this book and a group of women who strongly desire to lose weight and who will take a pledge to support one another and get together once a week. Pledges are important to your ability to stick with the program. A Dominican University of California study that examined the success of goal-setters found that those who wrote down their intentions were more likely to achieve them than people who merely made mental commitments.

Your club can be anything you want it to be, though we have a few suggestions to get you started. First, read the book before your initial get-together so you can discuss what you want to accomplish as individuals and as a group. There's much to discuss:

* Ways to increase your daily intake of the nutrient-dense foods featured in Chapter 4, as well as decrease the number of unhealthy foods in your diet

* How to change your habits around food and your attitude about food—an important aspect necessary to achieve permanent weight loss

* The best ways to keep and stick with a food diary, which studies show is the single-most-important tool for weight-loss success (see more on page 60)

* Coming to terms with the ways you undermine your own diet success, like giving in to a full-day binge when having just a slice of pizza would have satisfied your urge to eat

* The importance of putting yourself first and rewarding yourself so you can reach your weight-loss goal (see Chapter 7)

* How well you are doing incorporating the 10 life-changing weight-loss habits described in Chapter 3. For example, you might want to explore them one by one, a week at a time.

* Which activities you can do together that promote a healthier and more active lifestyle

* Recipes you'd like to try—you'll find nearly 100 recipes for breakfast, lunch and dinner in Part 2, The Girlfriends Meal Plan & Recipes

* Setting individual and group diet and fitness goals. Remember: Challenge yourself, but at the same time be realistic. A team goal depends on meeting your individual goal.

* Setting up a system of non-food-related rewards for members of your group

* Online diet websites that you could join as a team to compete with other diet teams

* Creating a Facebook page for your group to keep in contact between meetings and cheer each other on. Or setting up an email list or phone call chain for the group for when you feel yourselves weakening in resolve.

Don't worry if you don't get through all of these points in your first meeting. As long as you set your agenda for future meetings, you're sure to cover everything.

During your first meeting, do take some time to talk about your individual and team weight and fitness goals and what you might hope to achieve as a group. Then commit them to paper, sign and date. The individual pledge should include:

* Your weight-loss goal

* Your exercise goal

* Your commitment to support your sister dieters

* Your commitment to keeping a food journal

* Your commitment to attend weekly meetings—unless there is a circumstance equivalent to a doctor's excuse! Remember: Your success rate is tied to your commitment as a group.

YOUR INDIVIDUAL PLEDGE MIGHT READ SOMETHING LIKE THIS:

I want to lose 30 pounds so I can improve my health, renew my energy and be a good role model for my children. I will follow The Girlfriends Diet program of healthy eating and an active lifestyle, and support my girlfriends in achieving their goals. I will faithfully and honestly report what I eat and drink in my food diary and figure out my daily calorie intake. Being part of The Girlfriends Diet Club and attending its get-togethers is a high priority because I value my mental and physical well-being and what it will mean to my family.

YOUR TEAM PLEDGE—AS A PAIR OR A LARGER GROUP—MIGHT BE SOMETHING LIKE THIS:

We The [fill in your group name] Girlfriends Diet Club will support one another to achieve our individual goals, encourage those who stray, praise those who succeed, celebrate improving our health and maintain a positive attitude for all.

The key to permanent weight loss, as you will find out as you read on, is to change your relationship with food in a way that you can live with and *enjoy* day by day. To achieve *permanent* success, your weight-loss goal should be more than *I want to lose 30 pounds.* Your written goal should describe how you are going to achieve that 30-pound loss and your commitment to make sure those pounds don't come back.

FOR EXAMPLE:

My goal is to lose 30 pounds. I will strive to eat healthy each day by increasing my intake of vegetables, fruit and whole grains; limiting my intake of red meat; and avoiding sugar, refined grains and processed foods. I will limit my calories to _____ [fill in your number] and log a minimum of 10,000 steps on my pedometer every day. I also resolve to be more physically active in my daily life.

You can make your club more interesting, fun and accountable if you set a group weight-loss goal—the total of your individual commitments. Setting a predetermined weight-loss goal and achieving it is what keeps membership intact on the Trevose Behavior Modification Program, a successful volunteer-led group weight-loss program that's been in existence since 1970. Trevose believes that attending the weekly meetings is so important to the success of the group as a whole that missing a meeting can result in dismissal. You needn't go this far in setting up your rules, but it is important to emphasize that your club's strength and success rest on the individual commitment of all your members. The Trevose program and other experts also say that meeting weekly is best for motivation and accountability.

"I run with a group of women. It keeps us all on track."

—*Shari Stein,* Good Housekeeping *reader, Millburn, NJ*

To this end, at your first gathering, put your calendars together and pick your meeting times for the next two months. Mark them "top priority." After one month, look at your calendars again and schedule out another month. Meeting weekly is important to your success. Remember, you're all in this together, and success for everyone relies on each person's commitment.

Everyone needs to keep track of the calories they are consuming, and we'll tell you the important reasons why you want to do so on page 60. This can be done however you'd like—by hand in a pretty journal or online—but you must have access to your journal at every meeting of your Girlfriends Diet Club.

As for gadgets, you'll need a scale for a group weigh-in, if you choose to go that route, or if you prefer privacy, you can go by the honor system. We also recommend that each member get a pedometer. It's proved to be instrumental in achieving the exercise goals important to weight loss. In one large university-based study of women between the ages of 40 and 50, only those who religiously carried a pedometer each day increased the amount of walking they did throughout the day. And walking is the *minimum* amount of exercise recommended on this program. Any pedometer will do; they can range in cost from about $10 to $100. We like the Fitbit because it syncs with your computer and/or cell phone and allows you to work on individual and group goals.

FRIEND SOMEONE Friends don't matter just for the here and now; they matter for your future—your future *life*. Studies reveal that people with strong social networks live longer than those with less support. According to researchers at Brigham Young University in Provo, Utah, the positive effects of friends are comparable to—and this is a biggie—quitting smoking. Close family members and coworkers count toward this pal quotient, too. So why not invite your favorite work buddy for an after-work happy-hour glass of wine? Tell her it's doctors' orders!

Million-Dollar GF Advice for Getting Started

Big-budget movie studios have trainer Ramona Braganza on speed dial. Why? Because she's the pro at getting A-listers in amazing shape for filming. For now, she's a diet buddy focused on you. Here is her priceless advice that you can use to get started on The Girlfriends Diet:

1. Tell your friends you're trying to lose weight. "Many people think that trying to slim down is something they should keep private, so they rely on their willpower alone to stick to a program—and willpower only gets them so far!" Braganza says. Her client Jessica Alba, who has taken on several roles requiring her to wear skimpy clothing, sticks to a daily training and healthy-eating program with the help of friends and family, and entices them to work out and diet along with her. But you don't need to be cast in a movie to get

similar motivation and support: Declare your goal in your Girlfriends Diet Club or by posting it online where other dieters meet. "You want to connect with other women who are dealing with the same temptations—like couch time or cake—and staying on track."

2. Give yourself weeks, not days, to start seeing results. Fact: It's always better to train moderately than to try to do it all in a hurry, which is a recipe for burning out and giving up. "Remember Jessica Biel's fit-for-fighting body in the movie *Blade*? Well, she came to me a full two months before she started filming, so she didn't have to crash diet at the end and over-train," says Braganza. "Sound sane? That's the idea, and the key to not quitting."

3. Know what you're really eating—and not eating. Braganza has all her new

Are You Ready to Go, Girlfriend?

Are you ready to be a BFF to other dieters? To be the best friend that you can be to others, ask yourself these four key questions:

1. **HOW FED UP AM I ABOUT MY WEIGHT AND THE WAY I LOOK— REALLY?** When you're at the point where the pain of the present outweighs the sacrifice that change demands, you're ready—really.

2. **WHAT AM I WILLING TO GIVE UP?** "Cheating" is the dieter's downfall. Many women put themselves on a rigid plan, then cheat every chance they get. The Girlfriends Diet, however, is not about

clients keep a food diary that includes meals and all their components, timing of meals, portion sizes, water intake and exercise. "They find that things they didn't think were sabotaging their weight-loss goals actually are—like a daily latte and a couple glasses of wine," she says. "That can add an extra 500 calories a day! If you start shedding pounds but then hit a wall, this may be why." The good news is that it's possible to *double* your weight loss just by recording what you eat, some studies have found. Warns Braganza, "You can work out like crazy, but if you don't change your nutrition, you won't see results."

4. Walk like you've never walked before. You don't need to make starting up on exercise complicated. Braganza always recommends walking to her celeb-rity clients. "They love getting out for hikes or just strolling through their nabe with their dogs or babies," she says. She recommends beginning with 20 to 30 minutes three times a week, then building up slowly to five days a week. (We'll show you how in Chapter 7.) The best way to stay motivated: Wear a pedometer.

5. Use your brain to change your body. "The mind is a powerful weight-loss tool," says Braganza. Science backs this idea. One study found that thinking about the muscles you're using as you work them allows you to use more muscle fibers and build more strength. "Sometimes people rely on distractions like TV to get through a workout," she says, "but if you want to cut your workout time in half and slim down faster, focus on your body, not the tube."

sacrifice; it's about *adding* nutritious food to your diet and making a lifestyle change. To make it stick, though, you must expect to make the deal: You don't have to give up your favorite "fattening" foods forever, but you do have to commit to eating less of them less often. You also have to be willing to pick yourself up and start all over again when you stray.

3. AM I READY TO MAKE A COMMITMENT? Winging it doesn't work if you want to make a serious change in your life. You need to spell out clear, concise rules for yourself to eliminate ambiguity, and be

AMAZING! MAKEOVER! Vicki Baughman "*I lost 70 pounds—and found my new bff!*"

I'D ALWAYS BEEN a yo-yo dieter, but my weight struggles intensified after both of my sons were diagnosed with autism. I was so completely overwhelmed with caring for them that I forgot to take care of myself. I knew I had gained weight—I was wearing a size 28W—but it didn't hit me how bad it was until my husband snapped a photo of me on Christmas morning in 2007. As soon as I saw the image, I knew it was time to do something.

With my busy home life,

I knew I couldn't commit to a diet that involved a lot of planning and cooking. So I chose a planned diet that offered ease, convenience and pre-proportioned meals. I also started walking on a treadmill and spent time on message boards, where I made a lot of virtual girlfriends.

My husband committed to the diet along with me, which was great. Only for him it was easy. He lost 40 pounds, no sweat. But me? I was struggling with these crazy cravings! This is why meeting girlfriend

fellow dieters online became important to me. I think with women, dieting is much more of a mental thing. I met lots of women who were going through the same thing that I was. We challenged each other to stick to our diets and get more active. In a few months, I stopped relying on the pre-proportioned meals and I was finding that I was able to eat less and make healthier choices on my own. I was also down 20 pounds.

Online is also where I met Beth Hansen, who is

willing to share them with your diet buddies. They don't want to let you down; by the same token, you should be willing to commit to not letting them down.

4. **AM I READY TO BE ACCOUNTABLE?** It's easy to fool yourself into thinking you're on the straight and narrow when you're not. Establish a reality check that works for you. It could be a daily or weekly weigh-in. It could be changes in clothing size or keeping a photo of the original you at hand.

now my real-life best friend. We decided to do the Jillian Michaels *30 Day Shred* DVD together. We communicated every day and we compared notes along the way. Being accountable to my new friend, and having her support, made it much harder to quit.

In 14 months, I went from 186 pounds to 116 pounds, and I now wear a size 2. I'm happier, healthier and more active than I've ever been, which in turn makes my home life much more manageable. And it all happened in time for my 40th birthday! I have more energy to do the fun *and* hard stuff with my boys. But there's another great bonus: Beth. I live in Texas and she's in South Carolina, but we now get together in person. Also, we talk every day. Beth, who is five years older than me, is the person I call when I'm in the supermarket staring at a bag of cookies and I need someone to tell me why I should *not* buy them. She lost 55 pounds and looks fantastic. She's my inspiration. But I got help from a lot of other women as well. In fact, 15 of us got together for a giant girlfriends' weekend last year, and we're planning on doing it again. We're now real-life friends—all much happier in our skin.

"Being accountable to my new friend, and having her support, made it much harder to quit."

We'll get to the nitty-gritty of The Girlfriends Diet weight-loss and lifestyle program shortly, but first let's get in the face of some of the demons that make weight loss particularly challenging for women. Only by understanding the enemy can we figure out how to fight it.

Your GF Action Plan

MAKE A COMMITMENT TO CHANGE. The Girlfriends Diet is all about making a lifestyle change to a healthier way of living. Your first step is to *want* to lose weight and to *commit* to doing what it takes to get there.

FORM YOUR OWN DIET CLUB. You can follow The Girlfriends Diet as a solo pursuit but research shows that diets work best when you come together as a team. Form a Girlfriends Diet Club with friends, coworkers or other people in your community. Enlist a friend and buy her a copy at goodhousekeeping.com/girlfriends. Set up at least a month's worth of meetings, and make sure everyone has finished reading so that you're all on the same page. Then make it interactive by going online to keep in constant between-meeting contact with one another or to join other groups of like-minded dieters. Set up a private Facebook group or share your success on our Facebook page at facebook.com/girlfriendsdiet.

GET YOUR FRIENDS TO COMMIT TO YOU, AND MAKE SURE YOU COMMIT TO THEM. Realize that the success of your group hinges on the individual commitment and participation of each team member. Make sure to complete your individual and team pledges and goals at your first club meeting.

START TRACKING YOUR CALORIES. Before trying to change anything, spend a week eating what you normally eat and simply track your calories. At the end of the week, tabulate your calories—you'll use this information as you establish your dieting goals and calorie needs.

chapter 2 Women and Metabolism

WHAT WOMAN *HASN'T* BLAMED her weight struggles on her metabolism? *My metabolism is so-o-o slow! Losing weight was so easy in my 20s; now it just gets harder and harder.*

We blame our metabolism for our too-tight jeans, for the sad fact that we can't eat or party the way we used to and for the surprising reality that all our working out just doesn't seem to be helping us shed pounds. Most of all, we feel stuck, having to muddle through with the metabolism we've got. But just think for a moment: What do you really know about the "M" word—what it really means. Anyone? *Anyone?*

Getting in Touch With Your Metabolism

The relationship between you and your metabolism is a complicated one. You probably associate the word "metabolism" with weight gain and loss, but it's really the name for the process by which your body converts the food you eat into the calories you burn to fuel your daily bodily functions. Everybody has a Resting Metabolic Rate—what science calls your RMR—which is based on the amount of fuel (calories) it takes to get a body at rest through a 24-hour stretch. Eat just the right amount of calories to get you through the day, and you come out even in the end. The scale tomorrow morning should be what it was this morning. Eat less, and you'll burn off a little. Eat too much, and that excess fuel has to be stored somewhere—and, well, we know where that is.

Many people who are heavy and struggle to lose weight blame it on their metabolism—they think they were cursed with a slow burner. Not necessarily so. Just because you're overweight doesn't mean you have a slow metabolism—and, guess what, your skinny girlfriends don't necessarily have fast ones, either.

You might also presume that the bigger you get, the slower your metabolism will become, but that's just not the case. Overweight people actually tend to burn through calories more quickly because their muscles have to work harder to move those extra pounds. Of course, if you're more sedentary, as many overweight people are, you aren't engaging your muscles much, so your calorie expenditure is still going to be low.

Now for the real letdown. When you lose weight and get a little lighter, you need less food to fuel your daily needs. That's why it gets harder and harder as you continue losing weight—like you haven't noticed, right? Your RMR goes down because your body now needs fewer calories to function. A loss of up to 20 pounds can reduce your RMR by up to 70 calories a day, and 70 unused calories a day adds up to an extra seven pounds a year. You may be able to temporarily "trick" your metabolism into "speeding up" through some unsustainable calorie-starving fad diet—*no carbs! high protein! no fat!*—but once the diet ends, it all comes back to the basic fact of science

Could It Be Your Thyroid?

Probably not. Less than 12% of the population has hypothyroidism, a condition that meddles with all the chemical reactions in your body, including your metabolism, and that can lead to weight gain, among other symptoms.

And while it is true that certain medications for depression, bipolar disorder, and other mental conditions can lower your metabolic rate, experts stress that for the vast majority of us, it's our lifestyle choices—how much we eat, how little we move—that are to blame for a turtle-like metabolism and unwanted weight gain.

that has yet to be disproved: How much you weigh depends on the balance of calories eaten as food and calories burned for fuel. Eat more calories than you burn, and you gain weight—there's no way around it.

We wouldn't be telling you all this seemingly "bad" news if we didn't have a good reason—and the emphasis is on *good*. There is plenty you can do to get your metabolism working in your favor—*plenty*. Here's why: About 70% of your RMR is like a fixed cost. It goes toward the necessities of life, such as breathing, digestion, growing and repairing cells, and moving blood through your circulatory system. The other 30% is under *your* control. As researchers get deeper into the physiology of weight regulation, they are fine-tuning their understanding of what it takes to amp up that 30% and drop pounds.

Yes, our metabolism affects our size, how fast our personal motor runs and how efficiently we burn calories. But truth be known, a sluggish metabolism isn't the real reason we're packing on pounds. *We* are the reason. While the so-called speed of our metabolism is affected by such things as age, gender and hormones—things we can't control—the reason we gain weight has a lot to do with what we do, or don't do, with our body's calorie-burning machine. And that's something we *can* control, which we'll help you do starting on page 40 with our Metabolism-Boosting Strategies. But first let's take a look at the limits your age puts on your metabolism. It's a key factor in how efficiently you burn calories.

ADVICE FROM A BESTIE

The toughest part is getting to the starting line."

"I tell friends, 'Don't worry about making a perfect start, just start somewhere.' In my case, I spent four months calling the local gym to inquire about a membership before I finally walked through the door. Every week, the manager would phone me to say he hadn't seen me and try to get me to come in. When I finally did, he recognized my voice, gave me a big hug and said, 'It's time, isn't it?'

"I've weighed more than 300 pounds at three different times in my life. It got very depressing, and I stopped caring. But after my third child was born, I couldn't carry her up the stairs without getting short of breath, and I was having irregular heart rhythms. I knew if I kept going that way, I wouldn't see my kids grow up. I started by simply walking. At first I couldn't make it 500 feet without feeling exhausted, but every day, I took one more step. Then I would jog a couple feet, feel like I was going to die, stop and do it again.

"Eventually, I started working with a personal trainer—and little by little, I worked up to running a 10K. And I kept going! When I ran the Chicago Marathon for the first time, my sister called me every mile to cheer me on. When I was struggling, she asked me, 'Do you want to be fat for the rest of your life?' I said no, and she said, 'Then meet me at the finish line!' That's how I keep my momentum. I tell myself, 'You got to the starting line; that was the hardest part.'"

—*Kimee Armour, 43, Auburn, IL, who lost 175 pounds*

Fuel and the Female Body

It can happen at any age. You're eating what you want with no consequences. Then suddenly one day, it seems that one stray cookie and your jeans won't snap shut. According to Elisabetta Politi, R.D., nutrition director at the Duke Diet & Fitness Center in Durham, NC, beginning sometime in our 20s, we start burning fewer calories a day. And over the years, research has shown, it adds up to 10 calories a day; so each year you can gain about an extra pound—or 10 pounds in a decade—if you aren't careful! Other research has shown that a woman's metabolic rate falls roughly 2% to 3% each decade. A moderately active woman in her 20s requires roughly 2,000 to 2,300 calories a day to manage a healthy weight. In her 30s and 40s, it drops a little to just about 2,000. After 50, it falls to around 1,800. If you don't gradually adjust your diet over time, you can blow up to the next dress size all too easily.

Research suggests that even exercise in and of itself is not an antidote to age-related weight gain. New York–based fitness instructor and holistic health coach Craig Smith believes that the food you eat accounts for a full 85% of your body's appearance, while exercise dictates only the remaining 15%. "No workout will give you the results you want unless you change your diet, too," Smith says.

Most women's RMR can drop by 5% to 10% between their midteens and early 20s owing to a rise in reproductive hormones, says Jeffrey Morrison, M.D., a family doctor and nutritionist based in New York City. "As a woman enters prime childbearing years, estrogen, which increases body fat, rises," Dr. Morrison explains. At a cellular level, mitochondria, which convert glucose into energy, become less efficient, impairing the body's ability to burn fat and sugar. "As kids, our mitochondria work at full blast," says Oz Garcia, a New York City–based wellness and aging expert whose clients include Hilary Swank and Heidi Klum, "but they slow with age."

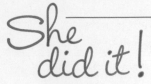

She did it!

LAURENE TENNANT-CHAVEZ
AGE **39**
LOST **17 POUNDS!**

HERE'S HOW: "My weight had been yo-yoing for a few years, but recently it had been more like a steady climb up the scale. I didn't want to buy new clothes, so I often wore stretchy leggings with a tunic. Even my wedding band didn't fit, and I wanted to be able to just slide it on again. And I wanted more energy.

"My *aha* moment was when my trainer at the gym told me that the formula for losing weight is 15% to 20% exercise and 75% to 80% nutrition. Before that, I was working out, but the scale wasn't budging. When I got real about how many calories I was eating—I kept a food journal on my phone—the pounds came off. I also had to retrain my brain. I kept telling my trainer, 'This body doesn't run.' So we started slow: just walking and doing 30-second spurts of jogging. Now I can run three miles—all thanks to my trainer."

Research conducted at the Cleveland Clinic shows that while portions of the human skeleton continue growing through the mid-20s, by her 30s, a woman's vertical growth has stopped and the hormones responsible for boosting muscle and bone strength drop off dramatically. Experts say these growth hormones also help prevent glucose absorption in fat cells, and when there is a deficiency, it's hard to lose weight. On top of that, these are the prime childbearing years. Pregnancy and breast-feeding mean many women temporarily increase their nutritional intake. It's also the age when chronic stress—brought on by full-fledged careers and family life—can cause overeating and trigger the release of cortisol, a hormone that signals the body to store fat around the midsection.

This is a time in your life when protein is especially important, says Dr. Morrison. He says he's seen patients become vegetarians only to find it harder to shed weight because they're consuming inadequate amounts of protein, which is necessary to maintain muscle mass and optimize metabolic function. Case in point? Jewelry designer Suzanne Somersall, 29, lost five pounds simply by cutting back on calorie- and carb-rich granola bars and by eating more lean protein like chicken, salmon and hummus.

As metabolism efficiency begins to drop further through the decades, your daily calorie requirements dip, too. In addition, women approaching menopause have less estrogen, meaning fat goes straight to the abdomen, instead of to the hips and thighs.

By the time you're in your 40s, overall health becomes a consideration along with your weight, and, experts say, you should consider them equally important. As you will learn in the next few chapters, you should be feeding your body heart-healthy fats like olive oil, which is actually easier to metabolize than butter, and antioxidant-packed and inflammatory-fighting fruits and vegetables, which can reduce the effects of chronic oxidative stress and illness. Meanwhile, Michael Moreno, M.D., a San Diego–based family practitioner and the author of *The 17 Day Plan to Stop Aging*, tells patients this age to start eating nuts, which have been found to possess life-extending compounds.

So, given *your* age, what is the magic RMR that will get you from the weight you are now to the weight you want to be? We're going to help you find out.

What's Your Calorie Burn?

Most of us know that if we want to lose weight, we need to swap out the pints of Chunky Monkey ice cream for chunks of apples. We also realize that portion size *does* matter. But if the way you're eating is making the scale go higher and higher, and cutting back isn't moving the scale, you need to get serious about counting calories. And that means knowing your personal RMR.

WISE FRIEND SAYS

Trimming 50,000 calories from your diet is ridiculously easy."

Really. Just replace one caloric drink a day—a soft drink or a vanilla latte—with water and it will save you about 50,000 calories in a year. That adds up to a 14-pound weight loss. And there's more: Swigging water won't just help you slash calories; it's a proven metabolism booster. Lesson learned: Drinks are treats, too, so sip wisely.

One of the most precise ways to determine your RMR is with a handheld calorimeter, which many gyms have. The device measures how much oxygen, which is used to create energy, you consume just breathing and provides a reading of how many calories your body requires each day. If you can't get your hands on a calorimeter, you can get a pretty accurate estimate of your RMR by using this scientific formula specifically targeted to women:

RMR=655+(4.35 x your weight in pounds)+(4.7 x your height in inches) - (4.7 x your age)

Now back in the old days when all we had to depend on were the three Rs, doing all this math might be a little much to ask. Now you can figure it out on your smartphone in less time than it used to take to dial a number (on an old landline). So jump on it.

Let's say you weigh 160 pounds (x 4.35 = 696) and you're 5 feet

5 inches tall (4.7 x 65 inches = 305.5) and you just turned 40 (x 4.7 = 188). So, 655 + 696 + 305.5= 1656.5 – 188 = 1,468.50 calories. In other words, at rest you burn roughly 1,470 calories per day. But even the most sedentary person will burn more than that just by smiling, laughing or fidgeting.

So now you need to factor in your activity level, which will increase your calorie burn by about 300 to 500 calories or even more, depending on how active you are. Choose the activity level that most closely describes you—be honest—and multiply your RMR by the factor indicated:

* Sedentary, meaning you do little or no exercise: RMR x 1.2
* Lightly active, meaning you do easy exercise or sports one to three times a week: RMR x 1.375
* Moderately active, meaning you do midlevel exercise or sports three to five times a week: RMR x 1.55
* Very active, meaning you do the equivalent of hard exercise or sports six to seven times a week: RMR x 1.725
* Extremely active, meaning you have a physically demanding job and get out there and exercise: RMR x 1.9

Using our example of a 40-year-old, 160-pound woman, being moderately active will boost her daily calorie burn rate to 2,276.

How Many Calories Do You Need to Lose Weight?

"It's simply a matter of intake versus output," says cardiologist Joseph Klapper M.D., author of *The Complete Idiot's Guide to Boosting Your Metabolism*. "Consume more calories than your metabolism needs, and you'll gain weight. Eat less and you'll lose."

Since a pound is equal to 3,500 calories, you would need to consume roughly 500 fewer calories a day to lose a pound a week.

There has been some refinement of thinking on this formula lately because everyone is different, but it is the equation science still holds onto as a general rule of thumb.

For faster weight loss, you can eat less, but don't be tempted to subtract too many calories. You don't want to consume fewer than 1,200 calories a day, warns Amy Jamieson-Petonic, R.D., spokesperson for the Academy of Nutrition and Dietetics. That will put your metabolism in starvation mode. As counterintuitive as it may seem, eating too little can slow your metabolism—by as much as 20%. "A body in self-starvation mode holds onto calories, so you're actually hurting, not helping, your metabolic rate," Jamieson-Petonic says. Not to mention the fact that there's no way your body can get all the nutrition it needs on such a severe calorie restriction.

If all this counting is not your bag, then start by limiting your calories to 1,400 a day—this amount is the basis of the menu plan (300 calories for breakfast, 500 calories for lunch and dinner, plus a 100-calorie snack or glass of wine) we created for The Girlfriends Diet. Your aim is to lose a pound or two a week. Apply common sense: If you're feeling hungry all day long or if you're losing weight at a faster rate than two pounds a week, you need to add 200-400 calories a day. If you have a lot of weight to lose, say fifty or more pounds, or if you are really active and burn more than 300 calories a day in exercise, then ratchet up your intake to 1,600 calories a day through meal snacks or additional sides. There are pointers on how to modify the meal plan on page 221.

Activity Boosts the Burn

Here is just a short list of how you can increase your calorie burn, based on a 160-pound woman, according to the formula used by scientists.

Activity	Duration	Calories Burned
Backpacking	4 hours	2,036
Golfing	4 hours	1,396
Dancing fast	1 hour	567
Resistance training	1 hour	536
Tennis singles	1 hour	530
Cleaning	2 hours	480
Actively playing with kids	1 hour	422
Skiing, downhill	1 hour	385
Running, 6-mph pace	½ hour	356
Pilates	1 hour	315
Yard work	1 hour	290
Jogging, 4-mph pace	½ hour	218
Swimming, low to moderate speed	½ hour	210
Hatha yoga	1 hour	181
Food shopping	1 hour	167
Stationary cycling, moderate speed	½ hour	127
Walking, brisk pace	½ hour	156
Walking, moderate pace	½ hour	127
Moving furniture around	15 minutes	105

Metabolism-Boosting Strategies

Metabolism is one of the most studied areas of weight-loss research. Scientists are continually looking for ways that will help give our resting metabolic rate a boost, all in the name of helping us lose weight. Here are some of the most ironclad strategies that you can use as you embark on The Girlfriends Diet:

BUILD MORE MUSCLE. It's an indisputable fact: Lean muscle burns calories more efficiently than fat. Every pound of muscle zaps six calories a day just doing nothing, while a pound of fat burns a measly two calories. The more lean muscle you have on your body, the faster your metabolism, the more calories you'll burn and the slimmer and trimmer you'll look. That's because even when your muscles are at rest, they still require three times more energy than fat does for tissue maintenance and rebuilding. "The best way to keep up your metabolic rate is by building muscle through physical activity and toning," says David Heber, M.D., Ph.D., director of the Center for Human Nutrition at the University of California, Los Angeles and author of *The L.A. Shape Diet*. Studies suggest that women can naturally lose up to 15% of their muscle mass before age 50. Women who work out to strengthen their muscles, on the other hand, can gain nearly three pounds of beneficial fat-free muscle mass in six months. Even if you gain a pound or so as a result of building muscle, it will still help your weight-loss efforts in the long run, because muscle stokes your metabolism. Plus, muscle takes up less room, so you'll look thinner. For the optimum metabolic burn, experts suggest that you:

* Get at least 30 minutes of cardiovascular activity most days of the week

* Do muscle-toning exercise at least two days a week

This doesn't mean you have to join a gym, or even that you have to do a straight half hour of cardio. Even everyday activities like walking, taking the stairs instead of the elevator or escalator, and gardening count toward your 30 minutes of cardio. "You can even squeeze in activity in 10-minute spurts through the day to see benefits," Dr. Heber says.

CURE SITTING SICKNESS. If you make phone calls for one hour at your desk, you'll burn 15 calories, but if you do it while standing up and pacing, you'll blast 100 calories. That's really NEAT—as in Non-Exercise Activity Thermogenesis—and ongoing research at the Mayo Clinic has found that we can burn up to an additional 800 calories a day simply by getting off our keisters and keeping our bodies moving throughout the day.

Not only does NEAT help drop pounds, but it also may have a greater impact on longevity than jumping around in a gym. A large study from the American Cancer Society found that women who sat for more than six hours a day were 37% more likely to die during the course of the next 14 years (while the research was ongoing) than those who were sedentary less than three hours a day. This association remained virtually unchanged even when the sitters were devoted exercisers. Keep this fact in mind when you read about ways to get moving in Chapter 6.

GET A GOOD NIGHT'S SLEEP. A single night of less sleep than the recommended seven to nine hours causes your resting metabolism to

---

She did it!

MILLICENT HOLCOMB
AGE **36**
LOST **19 POUNDS!**

HERE'S HOW: "When I got married five years ago, I was 146 pounds, but it wasn't a strong, toned 146. My goal when I started on my diet was to be fit, not just trim, and to look and feel even better than I ever had. There had been times when I'd showered with the lights off because I didn't want to step out and see myself in the mirror. I wanted my confidence back.

"When I first started dieting, I'd step on the scale four times a day. Today, I weigh in once a week. It's easy to become so focused on the numbers that you lose sight of everything else.

"Today, I'm stronger, healthier and happier, and everyone in my family has benefited. They helped me. They changed because I needed to change. I stopped cooking with butter—switching to only olive oil—and my husband and kids eat what I eat, mostly lean proteins and lots of veggies. We also started doing things together that are active but still fun; we've had a ball going roller-skating and rock climbing.

"Oh, as for the wedding dress? It is actually too big on me now!"

---

dip by about 5% the next day, says a study in the *American Journal of Clinical Nutrition*. "Sleep loss induces widespread hormonal changes that pump up the amount of ghrelin—the hormone that triggers appetite—in your body and dials down your metabolism," explains study coauthor Christian Benedict, Ph.D. So try conking out a little earlier for a better body and mood.

LOWER YOUR THERMOSTAT BY TWO DEGREES. When you're a little bit cold, your body has to work to generate heat to warm itself. One recent study found that people who spent time in a chilly room boosted their calorie burn by 80%. "Cold temperatures flip on the switch that makes your body burn calories like a furnace," says Scott Isaacs, M.D., an endocrinologist in Atlanta. And you don't need to sit there shivering: "Turning the thermostat down just a couple degrees can help you burn 100 additional calories a day," Dr. Isaacs says.

DRINK PLENTY OF WATER. Here's a reason to obey your thirst: "When you're dehydrated, cellular functions slow down and your metabolism starts to get poky," says Lauren Schmitt, a registered dietitian in Los Angeles. Yes, you can slim down just by drinking up. "People who down eight cups of water daily burn 100 calories more each day than those who drink four cups or less," says Schmitt.

MAKE BREAKFAST A MUST. Here's another finding: Breakfast eaters, for the most part, are thinner than breakfast skippers. Your calorie burn is at its lowest at rest. To wake it up and get it moving, you have to stoke it with energy—breakfast. Your metabolism slows while you sleep, and the process of digesting food in the morning revs it up. So don't leave home without it.

"Women mistakenly think they're 'saving' calories for later in the day, but they actually end up overeating and gaining weight," says registered dietitian Jamieson-Petonic. Studies show that breakfast eaters typically consume about 100 fewer calories per day than people who skip breakfast—that adds up to 10 pounds a year! This

AMAGING! MAKEOVER!

Jackie Freitag
"I lost 105 pounds—and ran two marathons."

I'VE BEEN A VEGETARIAN all my life, but I never liked vegetables. Instead, I lived off the "beige diet" of bread, macaroni and cheese, and peanut butter and jelly. I probably had a few extra pounds on me growing up, but my food choices really started to catch up with me in college. Even the aerobics classes I took twice a week weren't enough to balance out my snacking and nighttime eating. By graduation, I weighed 180 pounds and was a size 14.

It got worse. I drove to and from work, sat for eight hours at my job and collapsed in front of the TV at night. I'd eat two doughnuts for breakfast, grilled cheese and fries for lunch, half a box of pasta with butter and cheese for dinner, and I snacked on ice cream and chips while watching TV. My clothes became so tight that I wore stretchy yoga pants. My boyfriend, Eric, who'd always been fit, would suggest that we take a walk or bike ride, but I always came up with an excuse not to. I gained another 50 pounds. By September 2003 at age 26, I hit my peak at 230 pounds.

That month, Eric and I vacationed at Disney World. It was 90 degrees, and I was dripping with sweat. I was exhausted at the end of each day. I felt like a slug. One morning, Eric surprised me with breakfast at Cinderella's Castle, and we took a picture out front. I was wearing size 20 shorts and a men's size XL shirt. You'd think seeing a photo of myself that heavy would make me realize I needed to lose weight, but I thought, *That's a really good picture*. I was half hiding behind Eric, so you couldn't make out my double chin. We framed the photo and gave it to Eric's parents.

A few months later, I got the kick I needed. My friend Jill asked me to be the maid of honor at her wedding. Jill was thin, as were her other attendants; the thought of being the heavy one was horrifying. I had seven months before the wedding.

I began by eating healthier. I read that the average person eats 2,000 calories a day and that eating 1,500 calories could safely lead to weight loss, so I kept my daily calorie count between those two amounts. I experimented with foods like broccoli, asparagus, peppers, tofu and beans, and actually found out that I really enjoyed them. I kept track of everything I was eating in a food journal and found it empowering. I had cereal and orange juice for breakfast, organic frozen meals for lunch and energy bars as a snack. For dinner, I would eat a veggie burger, soup and salad, a vegetable omelet or one serving of pasta topped with tomato sauce. I also kept track of my calories and weight loss. Writing down what I'd eaten made me feel as if I was doing something good for myself. I went online and "talked" to other people who were going through the same thing. What a boost it was—and so motivating.

I also rejoined my old gym. This was really scary for me. I couldn't have been more wrong. But everyone was so support-ive—my old exercise buddies, my trainer. They were behind me, and I was psyched. By the time of Jill's wedding I was down 30 pounds. I remember putting on my dress and thinking, *I look pretty good*.

Since I was enjoying my routine, I kept at it. By March 2005, I wanted to try something new, so I ran

the short loop in my parents' neighborhood—about a third of a mile. I didn't even make it halfway before I had to stop and walk. A few days later I tried again. Eventually I made it! I starting running twice a week. Three months later, I was running three miles!

It was an exciting time, because I also got

"I kept track of everything I was eating in a food journal and found it empowering."

engaged. Besides the wed-ding, there was another event I had to look forward to—my first 5K. It was exhilarating to cross the finish line and have my parents and Eric cheering for me. By my wedding in August of 2006, I weighed 145 and felt perfect in my gown. Eric's first words were, "You look amazing!" I felt like my hard work

had paid off.

After the wedding, I signed up for a half marathon, and with all the training, I melted away another 20 pounds. In May 2007, the scale hit 125. I couldn't believe I had lost 105 pounds. Last year, I ran two full marathons.

Just after my 30th birthday, Eric took me to Disney World and said, "Want to retake that photo in front of the castle?" This time I was a size 4. We gave the new photo to his parents, who replaced the old one with it. Eric had always told me I looked good, even when I was heavy, but now we're able to experience more together. We go hiking and boating together now.

My goal going forward is to stay healthy and keep on racing. My mantra is, "Nothing can stop me now"—and considering how far I've come, I truly believe it.

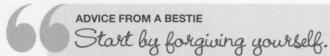

Start by forgiving yourself. "

"In November 2012, I hit 421 pounds, my heaviest weight ever. I'd tried pretty much every fad diet out there: Atkins, the grapefruit diet, pills. But my journey to better health really began when I changed my inner monologue from one that was negative and critical and said, *You're not worthy*, to one that said, *You can do this; you deserve to be healthy and happy and have love in your life.* I've had to forgive myself and be kind to myself in order to move forward—after all, I can't change what happened yesterday, but I can change what happens today and tomorrow.

"I started by signing up for a program that kept me accountable to a group of other dieters and by finding a pool I could use for exercise. Now the swimming pool is my second home. The water is so relaxing, like a cushion, and I can move without feeling hot or sweaty or straining my joints. I love it—it feels meditative.

"There's no way to shed the amount of pounds I have to lose and not be confused by the process at times. My weight has been such a part of my identity that losing it can feel overwhelming. Every day I have the opportunity to make choices about my health. Before, my eating and physical habits were thoughtless. Now, I pause and think before I decide to put something in my body or skip a workout. I still have a ways to go, but my goal isn't to be skinny; it's to feel better about myself, and I'm definitely on that path."

—*Elizabeth Agosto, 34, Hanover, NH, who lost 78 pounds and still counting*

doesn't mean you have to eat as soon as you roll out of bed. The sooner you eat after waking up, the better, but studies show that as long as you eat within three hours of getting out of bed, you'll reap the metabolic benefit.

GET A LITTLE PROTEIN AT EVERY MEAL. Eating protein at every meal, especially breakfast, is important for stoking calorie burn because it takes more energy to digest protein than it does to digest carbohydrates and fat. Plus, you need protein to build muscle. However, this does not mean that loading up on eggs and steak is the key to long-term weight-loss success. "You need carbohydrates and fat for energy, too," Jamieson-Petonic says. You can't live without them.

One study conducted in the Netherlands found that eating a healthy amount of protein helps you drop pounds and keep them off. So what's a healthy amount? The study authors suggest about half a gram a day for every pound you weigh. For the typical woman, that would be the equivalent of having an egg at breakfast, maybe a tuna fish sandwich for lunch, some cottage cheese as a snack and some chicken for dinner. Just don't overdo it. "Protein doesn't have any superpowers," says Felicia D. Stoler, D.C.N., an exercise physiologist. "Excess calories from protein will just get stored as fat." On The Girlfriends Diet, you'll be eating around 20% of your calories through protein.

GF Action Plan

FIGURE OUT YOUR CALORIE NEEDS. If you haven't already, use the RMR formula in this chapter to find your daily calorie needs and compare that with the amount of calories you are currently consuming. Check in with your Girlfriends Diet buddies and make sure they've figured out their current RMR and calorie intake numbers as well. In Chapter 3, you'll learn how to use this information as part of your diet plan.

START MOVING. Commit to getting out of your chair at work and off the sofa at home to do some sort of activity once an hour—it doesn't have to be long, but even walking around the block, pacing while you're on the phone with a girlfriend or marching in place during TV commercials will keep your metabolism moving faster, and burn extra calories along the way.

WISE FRIEND SAYS

Sip cold water to boost your burn."

Research shows that drinking two 8-ounce glasses of water can increase metabolism by 30%—and drinking cold water can boost the burn even more. So keep a glass on your desk, make frequent trips to the watercooler, and drink a glass with or before each meal.

If you find water is just too boring, spike it with vitamin C–rich lemon. Better yet, slice a lemon into your fridge's water jug and let it sit overnight. Another way to get a cold-watery boost: Sip unsweetened iced tea, which will also give you a shot of appetite-suppressing caffeine.

CHOOSE ONE OF THE METABOLISM-BOOSTING STRATEGIES for you and your Girlfriends Diet Club to focus on each week, and whether it's sleep, water or movement, commit to making it a priority until you meet again.

✱ Order a copy of *The Girlfriends Diet* for your friend at goodhousekeeping.com/girlfriends.

✱ Share your success stories and get more dieting tips on our Facebook page at facebook.com/girlfriendsdiet.

Weight Loss Never Tasted So Good

chapter **3**

BAGUETTES, BEANS, AVOCADOS, almonds, pasta, Greek salad—imagine a weight-loss diet that recommends you eat them almost *daily*. Now, look in the mirror and imagine yourself two, three or even more sizes smaller.

That's The Girlfriends Diet—follow it and one can lead to the other.

The Girlfriends Diet is different from other diets you have tried—and if you're like many of the girlfriends we know, that includes *a lot* of fad diets. You know, the kind you go on for as long as you can possibly stand it and, hopefully, drop a fast 10, only to feel the pounds creep back on. The Girlfriends Diet isn't an on-again, off-again kind of diet in which you eat this and not that, or avoid an entire food category (carbs! gluten!). Rather, The Girlfriends Diet is a collection of healthy eating *habits* based on the traditional Mediterranean diet, a *style* of eating that is widely believed to be the healthiest in the world.

Adopt them and you will discover a totally healthful and deliciously girl-friendly new style of eating—one you can enjoy and savor for a lifetime. Eating this way allows you to lose weight naturally, without gimmicks, at a healthy rate of about one to two pounds a week. It's designed so you'll never have to go on and off diets again because you'll want to continue to eat the same delicious foods on this plan. "The Mediterranean diet has long been accepted as an example of a well-balanced diet, but there is no gold standard 'Mediterranean diet,'" says Christiana A. Demetriou, Ph.D., a researcher in epidemiology and biostatistics in Cyprus. "At least 16 countries border the Mediterranean Sea, and diets vary between these countries and also between regions within the same country." However, Demetriou says, they all share common characteristics: high consumption of fruits, vegetables, bread and other cereals, potatoes, beans and nuts; low to moderate intake of dairy products, fish, eggs and poultry; and infrequent consumption of red meat. "In the Mediterranean diet, olive oil is frequently consumed and is an important monounsaturated fat source, and wine is consumed in low to moderate amounts," she says.

Defining "Classic"

The classic, or traditional, Mediterranean diet refers to the way of eating common to the regions of the Mediterranean Basin prior to the 1960s—*before* the people there were introduced to "American-style" meat and potatoes, convenience packaging and fast-food chains. Back then, overweight and obesity rates were low, but not today. Statistics and observational studies show that as more and more of the younger generations in the Mediterranean regions adopt Western-style eating habits, obesity rates are rising right along with them.

There's only one response to this way of eating, so let's hear it: *Yum!*

Your goal on The Girlfriends Diet is to adopt these same eating patterns and make them your new lifestyle—and when you form a group of girlfriends or diet buddies to do it along with you, you'll have each other's support to help make the changes permanent. "We know that healthier behaviors practiced among women become a pattern, and thus they can become a lifestyle that promotes health," says Cécilia Samieri, Ph.D., a researcher at the Université de Bordeaux in France and at INSERM, the French equivalent of the U.S. National Institutes of Health. Research shows that consistently trying to repeat a desired new habit for 30 days is about what it takes to make it stick.

You will be weaning yourselves away from a Western-style diet that is low in vegetables, fruits and whole grains, and instead modeling your eating after a Mediterranean-style diet, which is high in nutrient-packed vegetables, fruits, grains, legumes and other healthy foods. To help you get started on this new way of eating, Samantha Cassetty, M.S., R.D., developed the delicious recipes and meal plan you'll find in Part 2 of this book. They were specially created with busy women in mind and feature easy-to-find ingredients, no over-long prep or cooking times, and lots of taste appeal.

As this new style of eating becomes the focus of your diet, you will naturally drop to your ideal weight *and* reduce your risk of developing chronic health problems as you age—the two hallmarks that make the Mediterranean diet so famous.

Studies show that the Mediterranean diet more than any other program—including healthy ones—is easier to follow and produces the best chances for long-lasting results. That's because it is food-centric—it's all about flavor and enjoying foods that are filling by nature. And they are foods that are appealing to most women. In fact, when you convert to a Mediterranean diet and adopt it for a lifetime, your chances of relapsing and gaining your weight back "are almost nonexistent," said Lluis Serra-Majem, M.D., Ph.D., of the Mediterranean Diet Foundation.

Not so on other programs. A *JAMA* study that followed three well-known programs—Atkins (high-protein, low-carbohydrates), Ornish (vegetarian and low-fat) and Weight Watchers (calorie-restricted on a points system)—found that, after one year, they all produced only "modest" results and overall adherence rates were "very low." Similarly, another large, long-term study that spanned six years, randomly put 322 men and women on one of three diets: a low-fat, calorie-restricted diet (like Ornish); a low-carbohydrate diet without calorie restriction (like Atkins); and a Mediterranean, restricted-calorie plan (like you'll be eating on The Girlfriends Diet). All produced weight loss initially—about six pounds in the low-fat group, just over 10 pounds in the low-carb group and nearly 10 pounds in the Mediterranean group. But six years later, the low-fat group was within a pound of its original weight and the low-carb group was down only 3.7 pounds. The Mediterranean diet group, however, had retained a nearly seven-pound loss—what the researchers described as "healthy dietary changes" with "long-lasting, favorable" results.

Numerous studies have shown repeatedly that a diet that mimics the eating habits of people who live in areas of the Mediterranean consistently results in weight loss and prevents weight gain. "It is a valid dietary approach for losing weight and total body fat in particular," says Lee Hooper, Ph.D., a senior lecturer in research synthesis and nutrition at the University of East Anglia in Norwich, England. One specific study, also published in *JAMA*, found that 60 obese young women who followed a Mediterranean diet lost an average of *30 pounds* over the course of two years, and they weren't even really "dieting." They just adopted a healthier way of eating!

They were consuming *more* complex carbohydrates like fruits, vegetables, grains and legumes; *more* foods rich in monounsaturated fats, like olive oil; and *more* fiber. As a result, they were naturally eating *fewer* calories and *fewer* foods high in saturated fat. And they achieved what the study really set out to prove: Following a Mediterranean diet can improve two crucial conditions that compromise health. It lowered their insulin resistance, a condition that encourages the body to store fat and results in diabetes; and it reduced chronic inflammation, a leading contributor to heart disease, diabetes and cancer.

The "Magic" of Mediterranean

The evidence is strong: Eating a Mediterranean diet offers something that few weight-loss programs can—better health. Hundreds of studies have repeatedly found that people who adhere to a Mediterranean style of eating have a better quality of life—both physically and mentally. They have the lowest incidence of obesity, lower body fat, a lower risk of gaining weight and are less prone to chronic disease, and they are mentally sharper than people who eat a lot of processed meats and red meat, butter, margarine and sugar, reports the British medical journal *BMJ*.

"One of the most accredited hypotheses is that the Mediterranean diet is positively associated with better overall health status and reduced risk of major chronic diseases because of its high content of different beneficial compounds largely present in leafy vegetables, fruits, olive oil, red wine, fish and nuts," says Marialaura Bonaccio, a researcher with Catholic University of the Sacred Heart in Milan, Italy. Research suggests that the foods and the powerful antioxidant nutrients they contain work synergistically to fight the inflammation that leads to stroke, chronic illnesses such as heart

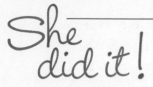

She did it!

JEANELL BOOMER
AGE **36**
LOST **14 POUNDS!**

HERE'S HOW: "Obviously, I need to lose weight—I'd love to just be out of the 200s!—but what's important to me is my health. I don't feel like the young 36-year-old that I am. I want to run around with my kids and not huff and puff. I love to dance—I'm making that a part of my exercise!

"I'm down 14 pounds—but still counting. It's just taking me awhile to get a handle on my eating habits.

"For example, I'd tell myself I had to eat things that weren't good for me because my family expected me to cook and bake certain foods—with no shortage of butter or oil. After I stopped the rationalizing, the weight started to come off. And it's true what they say: Once you lose the first 10 pounds, you really gain momentum."

disease, metabolic syndrome, diabetes, cancer and neurodegenerative diseases like Alzheimer's. Among the findings, eating a Mediterranean diet can result in:

LESS FAT AROUND THE MIDDLE. A study of nearly 50,000 people in Europe—70% of whom were women—found that adherence to a modified Mediterranean diet was associated with lower abdominal fat, according to the *Journal of Nutrition.*

REDUCED RISK OF BREAST CANCER. Diet has long been suspected to have an impact on breast cancer risk, and a Mediterranean diet has been associated with a lower risk of cancer in general. Now a study has found a link between eating a Mediterranean-style diet and a reduced risk of breast cancer. The study, published in *BMC Cancer,* followed the dietary habits of 1,700 women in Cyprus, a country where the incidence of breast cancer is low. "Our results suggest that adherence to a diet pattern rich in vegetables, fish, legumes and olive oil may favorably influence the risk of breast cancer," says Demetriou, the lead researcher on the study.

BETTER CONTROL OF BLOOD SUGAR. One of the most promising findings in the Mediterranean diet's healthfulness is its apparent ability to help reverse insulin resistance, a condition in which the body cannot adequately regulate the release of glucose during digestion. Insulin resistance is a major health concern because it is believed to contribute to obesity and can lead to diabetes.

When insulin function is compromised, theories suggest, the body does not adequately convert fat into energy and instead stores it in cells. Several studies show that when people with insulin resistance (also known as prediabetes) convert to a Mediterranean diet, insulin regulation improves. The reason? The foods eaten on the Mediterranean diet typically scale on the lower end of the glycemic index, meaning they release glucose slowly so insulin doesn't have to work overtime.

DIMINISHED SYMPTOMS OF METABOLIC SYNDROME. Several studies have found that the inflammatory-fighting effects of the Mediterranean diet reduced the symptoms in people with metabolic syndrome, a cluster of conditions (high cholesterol, high blood pressure, overweight and diabetes or prediabetes) that increase the risk of heart disease. One study, reported in the journal *Obesity*, found that fol-

The Way to Shed "Baby" Fat

An estimated 15% to 20% of pregnant women retain 10 or more pounds of their "baby weight" after delivery, increasing their risk of obesity and the chronic conditions that go with it. They are also in a persistent state of chronic inflammation. However, according to a study conducted at the University of Arizona, a Mediterranean-style diet can be the antidote to both problems. In the study, breast-feeding women who ate a healthy Mediterranean diet shed six to 7½ pounds of excess weight over a four-month period and experienced a reduction in inflammation—just by eating healthy!

lowing the diet even in the absence of weight loss "significantly reduces inflammation" associated with the condition.

BETTER QUALITY OF LIFE AS YOU AGE. Women who followed the healthy eating patterns of the Mediterranean diet were 40% more likely to survive to age 70 and beyond without experiencing major health problems, physical impairments or mental decline, according to the long-term Nurses' Health Study, which followed the eating habits of more than 10,000 women. "The women who ate healthier not only lived longer, but they also thrived," says Cécelia Samieri, who led the research for Harvard Medical School and Brigham and Women's Hospital in Boston. They also were more likely to be classified as "healthy agers," she says. Although Samieri did not study how long someone has to be on the diet to garner these benefits, she says, "Adopting it earlier rather than later is probably better."

The Gender Gap

When British researchers went on a quest to find the differences in the way that men and women look at food, they found that men really do have a meat-and-potatoes mentality. "One of the most striking findings was that women tend to favor healthier meals in that they rated them higher on dimensions of pleasure, convenience and health than did men," says Cheryl Haslam, one of the study's researchers and a professor of health psychology at Loughborough University in Leicestershire, England. "Women also tend to have higher levels of health knowledge. They are more likely than men to report declines in meat consumption and less likely to see meat as important to healthy eating."

Even though obesity rates are similar between men and women, "Women are more willing to be engaged in attempts to lose weight," says Haslam. Cutting back on calories and eating healthy foods are just things we are programmed to do.

So in many ways, women are already poised to follow a Mediterranean style of eating. All you need are the directions—and we've got them for you right here.

So, let's get started. Repeat after us: *The Girlfriends Diet is not just a diet; it is a lifestyle.* It's the change you're going to make to lose weight, get healthier and feel more energetic.

You'll lose weight on it because you're going to eat fewer calories than you burn until you reach the weight you want, but you'll want to stick with it forever because you'll develop a taste for it—just like the millions of people in the Mediterranean regions who can't imagine eating any other way. You will succeed in your weight-loss attempt because teaming up with friends to diet along with you and/or enlisting a support group will help keep you motivated and make you feel accountable to others.

"A Mediterranean-style eating plan," explains Marta Garaulet, who designed The Garaulet Method, a program based in Spain that combines a Mediterranean diet with professionally directed nutritional and behavior therapies, "is really appealing to women because they really love the food on it, so they adapt well." And so will you. "It is a lifestyle because it has well-recognized nutritional benefits and high taste appeal suitable to social and daily life. It's just a natural way of eating, so it can be adopted for a lifetime," Garaulet says.

The Girlfriends Diet follows all the healthy principles of a Mediterranean diet while restricting enough calories to result in a one- to two-pound weight loss a week. It is achievable and sustainable because:

* It is highly satisfying, owing to its high fiber and high fat content

* It is surprisingly high in the amounts of food you can eat because it is composed largely of fruits and vegetables

* Its high-carbohydrate content means it does not trigger specific cravings that can lead to binge eating

✳ In spite of being calorie-limited, it offers healthy amounts and a variety of antioxidants and other important nutrients

It is structured around these daily goals:

✳ Consuming in the range of 1,400 to 1,600 calories a day, but never fewer than 1,200 calories a day to lose weight. This amount is based on your reducing your current daily calorie consumption by 500 to 1,000 calories a day and is your daily calorie allotment that you'll use while losing weight.

✳ Having three full meals a day totaling 1,300 calories: 300 calories at breakfast and 500 calories each at lunch and dinner. In addition, you can have one snack or glass of wine on the 1,400-calories-a-day program, or 300 calories' worth of snacks including a glass of wine on the 1,600-calories-a-day plan. However, you may be able to eat even more and still lose weight, depending on how active you are. (See page 37.)

✳ Eating the majority of calories before midday (3 P.M.), if possible, and all meals before 8 P.M.

✳ Consuming 50% carbohydrates, 20% protein and 30% total fat, with no more than 10% of calories coming from saturated fat

✳ Aiming to use olive oil as the primary added fat

✳ Eating a mostly plant-based diet with a little protein at every meal. This means getting at least 50% of calories from fruits, vegetables, whole grains, and legumes including unrestricted amounts of vegetables (a minimum of seven ounces a day) and fruits (at least eight to 10 ounces a day).

✳ A minimum of 30 grams of fiber, which is easily achieved by eating this way

Once you lose the weight you want all you have to do is figure out the number of calories you need each day to sustain your new weight using the RMR formula in Chapter 2. Most women will be able to maintain their weight by eating 1,800 to 2,200 calories a day depending on how active they are. That's the beauty of The Girlfriends Diet — there are no "diet" foods you must eat or foods you must do without. The only difference is that once you lose the weight you want, you can continue to eat more of the same delicious foods.

Making This Lifestyle a Habit

The Girlfriends Diet is not just a weight-loss program; it is a lifestyle based on the habits that make the Mediterranean diet so healthy. We've condensed them into 10 goals, or what we're calling Girl-Friendly Habits. These 10 habits are the keys to eating in a way that will help you lose excess weight naturally and keep it off for a lifetime.

Forming a new habit takes practice, as we noted in Chapter 1. If you already eat a mostly healthy diet, adjusting to this style of eating may be easy. You'll take to it like a fish to water. If you don't eat a lot of vegetables and fiber, are a fast-food junkie or eat a lot of red meat, it might take you some time to adjust, so don't expect to take to it overnight. This is where your diet club can be helpful. Your girlfriends are there to encourage you and offer you their own experiences and advice.

One proven way to help adjust to a new style of eating is with a little cognitive therapy, says Garaulet. You want to train your mind to keep you focused on these habits. A good way to start is to write down these 10 habits and keep them front and center so they become instilled in your daily thought processes. Post them where you can see them—attach them to your bathroom mirror as a reminder when you brush your teeth in the morning, or design them as your computer-screen wallpaper.

Another, even more important, way is to keep a food diary. Research has found that keeping a food diary is the single-most-important weight-loss tool. You should write down everything—what you eat, when you eat, where you eat, what you were feeling or thinking at the time. It helps you identify triggers that make you eat out of habit. Identifying those triggers is the way to start learning how to avoid them. A lot of research supports this conclusion, so make sure that you are keeping track of your meals and calorie intake.

Discussing the following 10 habits should be a part of your weekly Girlfriends Diet Club meetings. Ask everyone how they're doing, what innovative ways they've found to keep on track, what their daily challenges are. Be open about your stumbles and achievements. Remember, you're in this together. Keep practicing, and these new habits will become second nature and healthy eating will naturally fall into place.

GF Habit No. 1 » *Count your calories*

As you well know, losing weight is a matter of arithmetic—calories in versus calories out. Eat fewer calories than you burn, and you'll lose weight. Eat more, and you'll gain. There's no getting around this scientific fact. The RMR you figured out on page 36 is the number of calories required to keep you at your *current* weight. Cut back 500 calories a day, and theoretically you should lose a pound a week. If you cut back 800 calories a day, you will theoretically lose about 1½ pounds a week; 1,000 calories, two pounds. We say "theoretically" because everyone is different. How fast or slow you lose weight depends on a lot of variables, like your age, how much weight you need to lose, your activity level, how severely you are cutting calories and how efficient your metabolism really is.

Typically, weight loss can start out a little faster, mostly because you're getting rid of water weight; then it may slow down. You might also go for a week or more without losing *anything*—that all-too-well-known plateau we all hear about. Discouraging, yes, but we encourage you to keep plugging away because negative caloric intake will cause weight loss. In the end, it should average out.

According to weight-loss experts, a good, healthy weight loss is anywhere from a half a pound to two pounds a week, depending on how heavy you are starting out. So if you are trying to lose 20 pounds, for example, it should take you between two to four months. Also remember: Don't go below 1,200 calories a day. Not only can it slow your metabolism, but you're also putting yourself at risk nutritionally. Any nutritionist will tell you that it is difficult to get your minimum daily requirements of all the essential nutrients if you eat fewer than 1,200 calories.

Also keep in mind that various gadgets and apps can help track your progress. A pedometer measures the steps you take each day and how many calories you burn. Pedometers are proving to be great motivators in getting people to burn more calories through walking. There are also electronic programs you can download on-line for free to your smartphone or computer that work in the same way. Some gadgets, such as the popular Fitbit, which retails for $60 to $100, can do it all for you.

GF Habit No. 2 » Know your carbs

It's been more than 40 years since carbs became the big no-no among dieters, and no matter how often and how vigorously this has been disproved, women are still living in fear of carbs.

Well, we're here to tell you emphatically: *Let it go!* We *need* carbs. We can't live without them. On The Girlfriends Diet, you're going to devote from one-half to three-quarters of your plate at every meal to carbohydrates. That's right. The Girlfriends Diet is decidedly carb-centric.

"Women need carbohydrates because eating them helps us maintain high serotonin levels, the brain chemical that signals that we are full," says Garaulet. Serotonin is our satiety button. "Women naturally have less serotonin than men. On a high-protein diet, it is not easy to maintain serotonin levels. Low serotonin levels are related to the carbohydrate craving that is frequently associated with obesity."

Before you put your hand in the cookie jar, be aware that the task at hand is knowing which carbs you can eat. "Not all carbs are created equal," reminds Joy Bauer, R.D., founder of Joy Bauer Nutrition Centers and the nutrition expert for the *Today* show. There's a difference between load-your-plate, good-for-you carbohydrates and the get-your-metabolism-into-trouble, bad-for-you variety. Obviously—no surprise!—your goal is to reach for the good and avoid the bad.

Good carbs are the complex kind that we find in deliciously crunchy whole grains and fill-your-mouth-with-flavor asparagus, spinach and other low-cal vegetables. These are the foods that define the Mediterranean diet. Then there are the bad carbs—what are referred to as simple, or refined, carbs. They are usually easy to identify because of their *tsk-tsk* color: white. That includes anything made with white flour and sugar. Refined carbs offer little in the way of nutrition and get broken down by your body and used quickly, says Bauer. "When you eat them, you may get a temporary burst of energy, but you'll inevitably feel tired or hungry again soon after."

Complex carbs do just the opposite. Your body breaks them down much more slowly, so you'll feel fuller longer. It's why we can eat fewer calories on a Mediterranean-style program and not feel hungry. What's more, high-quality carbs come packed with important nutrients—vitamins, minerals, antioxidants and fiber. Eating this way also ensures that you automatically get adequate fiber intake—at least 30 grams each and every day. There is no reason to count fiber.

Vegetables and fruits are the best diet-friendly carbs. Other carbs to love, but only in moderation, are starchy veggies like potatoes, corn and peas. Grains are also great for you—but their starchiness packs in more calories. So be careful when choosing them so you don't go beyond your daily limit. Portion sizes for all of these are half a cup.

Nothing is more important for losing weight than reaching for fruits and vegetables throughout the day, says Bauer, but that isn't the *only* reason you should eat them. Eating lots of produce is essential to lowering your risk of just about every ailment—especially cancer and heart disease—and staying at a healthy weight.

If eating *a lot* of plant food at each meal is new to you, here are some girl-friendly suggestions that work:

TAKE IT ONE SERVING AT A TIME. If you don't get much in the way of produce in your diet now, work up to it gradually. It may make the weight come off more slowly at first, but your primary concern is to make plant food the major source of your diet. "You'll be ahead of the curve if you just make sure to include at least one veggie or fruit at every meal," says Madelyn Fernstrom, Ph.D., author of *The Real You Diet*. It's something you can truly accomplish anywhere. It even works at fast-food joints. Order a side salad, baked potato or apple dippers instead of fries.

PUT SOUP ON THE MENU. Minestrone is a classic Italian Mediterranean soup. In some parts of Italy, people eat it almost every day. There are numerous styles of minestrones, so start experimenting with The Girlfriends Diet recipe on page 248. Minestrone makes a great light dinner. Add a grainy slice of bread and a piece of fruit, and you're set. Is chicken noodle more to your liking? Add fewer noodles and in their place throw in an assortment of vegetables. In fact, you can add veggies to just about any of your favorite soup entrées. Get creative. It's a great way to use up vegetables you have in the fridge that are approaching their expiration date.

MAKE YOUR PLATE A COLOR CHART. When you pile your plate high with veggies, strive to include the important colors of orange/red (squash, berries and tomatoes, for example), black/blue (eggplant,

Plan a Week in Advance

The biggest problem women have feeding themselves well? They're too busy. We have that enabling need to take care of others and others' needs first—including their need to eat healthy. Even professional health foodies have a hard time eating right all the time. "When my three kids were little and I was traveling a ton, I needed a way to make cooking healthy meals and snacks easier," says Kathy Kaehler, a food coach and celebrity trainer. She started prepping a week's worth of veggies, proteins and grains on Sundays so she could throw together yummy pastas, salads or rice dishes in minutes on busy weekdays. Now she teaches her 90-minute routine, which she calls "Sunday Set-Up," to clients like the Kardashians and has an online club dedicated to it (kathykaehler.net/club).

It's so simple and brilliant, you won't believe you haven't always done this. Each Sunday:

1. CHOOSE four to six veggies, two to three proteins and two whole grains. Example: Broccoli, bell peppers, carrots, Romaine lettuce and other firm-textured veggies keep well. Chicken breasts, eggs and beans make for great go-to proteins. Brown rice and quinoa are versatile grains.

2. RINSE, CHOP, PREP. Bake the chicken and boil the eggs, rinse the canned beans, wash and chop the veggies, and cook the grains. Pop everything into clear containers and store in the fridge.

3. EAT! Pick your main ingredients and mix with dressings and add-ins to create dishes like Cobb salad, stir-fries or veggie pasta—plus snacks like peppers with hummus, or egg salad.

blueberries) and white/yellow (corn, zucchini, cauliflower, etc.), and, of course, the vast assortment of green and leafy greens. Not only does it make your plate look appealing, but you'll know you're getting your fill of the anti-inflammatory antioxidants that make the Mediterranean diet so famous. (You'll read all about the bounty of nutrients in Mediterranean foods in Chapter 4).

DROWN YOUR ENTRÉES WITH VEGGIES. When Penn State University researchers substituted a vegetable puree for 25% of an otherwise ordinary main course (macaroni and cheese, or chicken and rice, for instance), they found that study participants nearly doubled their vegetable consumption and ate on average 357 fewer calories over the course of *a day*. Best of all, despite the mega drop in calories, they pronounced the entrées as delicious and reported feeling as full afterward as they did when they ate at liberty.

EAT YOUR VEGGIES FIRST. Evidence suggests that if you eat the lower-calorie items on your plate first, it will help take the edge off your hunger and you'll be less likely to overeat. A study at Penn State also found that people who doubled up on vegetables and fruit in a meal saved calories overall.

TRY SOMETHING NEW EVERY WEEK—OR MORE OFTEN. It's another thing your mother was right about: You'll never know if you like something unless you try it. Weight problems can have many causes, and eating the wrong kinds of foods is high on the list. Some people defend those choices by saying that they just don't like vegetables. But when was the last time you tried a new way of eating spinach or tasted an exotic grain like quinoa? Don't like steamed broccoli? Try it roasted, or sauté it with garlic.

For most people, losing weight means replacing calorie- and fat-laden foods with new ones. Make it a habit to pick up something new in the produce section every time you food shop and give it a try. More than likely, you'll be discovering a new, diet-friendly food.

Cut Back on Processed Foods

Or, better yet, cut them out entirely. A Harvard study found that dieters who followed a weight-loss plan based on healthy, unprocessed carbohydrates such as fruits, veggies and whole grains, instead of processed carbs, burned on average about 80 more calories a day—that adds up to eight pounds a year—than those who didn't. The reason: Less-processed foods tend to have less sugar, so levels of insulin, a fat-storage hormone, remain steady. Sugary processed foods, on the other hand, trigger a spike in insulin, which cues your body to hold on to fat.

Chapter 4 features 42 foods—mostly veggies and fruits—that are part of a Mediterranean-style eating plan. Get familiar with them all, and you'll find that your diet will never get boring.

GO VEGETARIAN ONCE OR TWICE A WEEK. Swap vegetables for meat just once a week, and you could drop four pounds in a year without changing anything else. When Johns Hopkins researchers fed 54 men and women similar lunches—one mushroom-based, the other meat-based—the veggie-based eaters consumed roughly 30 fewer grams of saturated fat than the meat eaters. And they reported that the vegetable-based meal was just as satisfying as eating meat. If you're a burger lover, all it takes is switching to a veggie burger.

GF Habit No. 3 » Cut the butter and add olive oil every day

Here's some news to make you smile: Fat isn't the villain it's cracked up to be. The Mediterranean diet, in fact, is *the* shining example. No one can say the Mediterranean diet is low in fat. That's because people who live in the Mediterranean Basin love olive oil. You could even say they consume it with abandon. In 2013 a study in the *New England Journal of Medicine* made major headlines when it reported that a healthy diet fattened up with olive oil reduced heart attack risk by 30% in a large group of aging Europeans possessing major risk factors. The fat they were adding to their diet was extra-virgin olive oil, and they were downing, on average, *4 tablespoons* a day!

There is a very important distinction in this delicious news: Olive oil is very different from butter, the typical American fat of choice, because it is healthy. It is teeming with heart-healthy artery-friendly monounsaturated fat, while butter is almost all health-robbing saturated fat. So while a Mediterranean diet may be higher in fat— great for its taste appeal!—it is still low in saturated fat, which is terrific for our health.

On The Girlfriends Diet, your goal is to make olive oil your fat of choice and whenever possible to minimize or eliminate your butter

WISE FRIEND SAYS

Forget reduced-fat foods. When you want something with fat, go for the real thing."

Fat-free may sound like the healthy choice, but it is actually less nutritious. "Fat-free foods often contain chemically based fake fats, which your body doesn't digest all that well, or extra sugar, which can spike your blood sugar and make you hungrier," says Karen Klimczak, R.D., of Mindful Nutrition Counseling in Chicago. "Eating some fat is also important because it helps you feel satisfied, so you're more likely to eat less."

Full-fat treats can satiate you more psychologically as well. In one study, when people were told they were drinking a low-fat milk shake, they said they felt less satisfied than when they were handed an "indulgent" shake, even though the two drinks were identical.

When trying to watch your calories and fat intake, choose low- or reduced-fat versions of foods you eat daily—yogurt, cheese and granola. But when it comes to occasional treats—a scoop of ice cream or one of your favorite cookies—go for the real thing. Just make sure you keep the portion small and the occasion rare. For example, a fist-size scoop of ice cream or a cookie that fits comfortably in your palm is as far as you should go.

intake. You want to eat olive oil daily not only because of its healthfulness, but because studies show it has a high satiety quality. Getting the right amount of fat—30% or less of your calories from total fat and 10% or less from saturated fat—is no problem when you use the meal plan in this book, because it's designed to make your overall intake fall within that range.

The fact still remains, however, that fat contains more than twice the calories of protein and carbohydrates—nine versus four calories per gram. And olive oil has more calories per tablespoon than no-no, not-on-this-diet butter—120 versus 100. So, how does that fit into a calorie-cutting plan? Apparently, our bodies respond better to olive oil than they do butter. It's easier to metabolize than butter and other saturated fats, so we burn it off faster. Australian researchers reported that people who were allowed to eat what they wanted for 12 weeks, so long as their diet was high in monounsaturated fats like olive oil, did not gain excessive weight. The reason: Olive oil on a Mediterranean diet is almost exclusively paired with low-calorie foods, such as leafy greens and other vegetables.

Interestingly, there seems to be a slight advantage to adding a bit of olive oil to vegetables. Reasearch shows that you need some fat on your salad or vegetables in order to absorb all their important anti-oxidants. Just make sure you use measuring spoons, as a little slip can make the calories add up fast.

GF Habit No. 4 » Get a little protein at every meal

The major difference between American-style eating and the eating customs of people who live in regions of the Mediterranean? Protein. Americans see it as the star of the meal—steak and mashed! In the Mediterranean, it is the accent. Your goal on The Girlfriends Diet is to do likewise. Picture a plate half filled with vegetables—spinach, asparagus, a little potato, a sliver of avocado, maybe—and the other side filled with a grain, such as couscous, a spoonful of beans and a bit of meat. This should be your goal at every meal.

Accenting each meal with a little protein is important as it will help you avoid the siren of the 9 P.M. ice cream or chocolate craving. According to a study in the journal *Obesity*, dieters who ate three meals a day and got 25% of their calories from protein felt 50% more satisfied and had 51% fewer late-night cravings than those who ate less protein. That's because protein triggers the release of the fullness hormone peptide YY, which tells your brain you're done eating, says study lead author Heather Leidy, Ph.D. Plus, protein takes longer to digest than carbohydrates, so it sticks with you.

There is a place in your diet for meat—poultry (chicken and turkey), pork and especially fish are all welcome on The Girlfriends Diet. Fish is especially important because it is our primary source of heart-healthy omega-3 fatty acids. You should have at least two servings a week, but eat it more often if you'd like.

There isn't much room on a Mediterranean diet for red meat, especially beef, because people in these regions traditionally don't eat a lot of it, mostly because it is not readily available. To be true to the Mediterranean style of eating means you should eat red meat on occasion, not more than once a week. However, if red meat is your thing, you don't have to give it up. A few servings a week are OK as long as you still eat your vegetables and grains and have enough calories left over to fit in the extra servings of protein.

Variety in your protein choices will help make your diet interesting and satisfying, says Monica Reinagel, M.S., L.N., a nutritionist

WISE FRIEND SAYS

Eat some fat at breakfast to boost your metabolism."

Research has found that incorporating fat into your wake-up meal turns on your fat-burning switch and helps your body use more calories all day long. Try this:

* 1 egg and ½ c. baby spinach cooked in 1 tsp. oil, and topped with 2 tsp. feta cheese; ½ whole wheat bagel thin spread with ¼ med. avocado: **277** calories

* 2 Tbsp. almond butter spread on a sliced apple: **293** calories

* ¾ c. plain nonfat Greek yogurt layered with ½ c. blueberries and ¼ c. walnuts: **311** calories

in Baltimore. "Pork and beef tenderloin, and flank steak are all quite lean," she says. By the same token, it's not necessary to avoid dark-meat chicken. Dark meat is a rich source of taurine, an amino acid that may help decrease heart disease risk in women with high cholesterol, according to a study conducted at the New York University School of Medicine.

Also, keep in mind that protein isn't all about meat. Strive to add plant protein to your plate, too, such as beans, soy, nuts—or else an egg.

GF Habit No. 5 » *Don't skip meals, especially breakfast*

Three squares a day, plus two snacks. That's the Girlfriends eating mantra—even if you're not feeling particularly hungry. Researchers at the Fred Hutchinson Cancer Research Center followed 123 dieters for a year and found that those who didn't skip meals lost eight more pounds than people who tried to speed up their weight loss by skipping meals.

Research has proved that successful dieters are eaters. They eat breakfast, lunch and dinner, and have a little something in between so they don't go down the slippery slope and show up at *any* eating occasion famished. Skipping meals is simply a weight-loss strategy that's sure to fail. Your own dieting history probably can tell you that!

A study at Virginia Commonwealth University found that dieters were able to lose impressive amounts of weight—23 pounds over four months, and another 17 pounds over the next four months—simply because they didn't bypass meals.

The problem with meal-skipping is that the one we're most likely to pass up is breakfast, and that's the worst one to ignore. Breakfast is essential to keeping our metabolism in peak performance. "Your metabolism slows while you sleep, and the process of digesting food in the morning revs it up," says Christine Gerbstadt, M.D., R.D., a spokesperson for the Academy of Nutrition and Dietetics.

Eating breakfast gives your diet a winning edge. Research shows that when the day is done, breakfast eaters typically consume about 100 fewer calories a day—that adds up to 10 pounds a year!—and weigh less than breakfast skippers. A British study of 6,764 people found that breakfast skippers gained twice as much weight over the course of four years as breakfast eaters.

Eating breakfast also is key to helping keep the weight off. When experts from the University of Colorado Health Sciences Center surveyed more than 3,000 successful dieters who had lost 30 pounds or more and had kept it off for at least a year, they found that eating breakfast was the one common denominator all the dieters shared.

The reason? "People who skip breakfast are more likely to snack impulsively during the morning," says Joan Salge Blake, R.D., clinical associate professor at Boston University. That makes you susceptible to what's available around you, like the doughnuts on the conference table at your staff meeting.

What Would a Nutritionist Do?

You make your 8 A.M. flight on an empty stomach. The only option on board: doughnuts. Caught between two bad choices—indulge or skip breakfast entirely—what would a nutritionist do?

"Eat the doughnut. Something is better than nothing. But avoid added sugar—jelly filling, sprinkles, frosting—and scrape off the toppings, if necessary. Best would be a plain doughnut sprinkled with nuts, plus a glass of milk to get in some protein and avoid a sugar crash."

—Angela Lemond, a Plano, TX, R.D. and
Academy of Nutrition and Dietetics spokesperson

For many breakfast skippers, though, running out the door on empty has nothing to do with some heroic diet ploy. They simply aren't hungry. But the "eat breakfast" rule does not mean you must eat the moment you roll out of bed in the morning. While it's better to eat as soon as possible, as long as you eat within three hours after rising, you will reap the metabolic benefit. Oatmeal, fruit, a piece of grainy bread—anything will do over nothing. Coffee alone, however, will not do the trick. Your goal should be to get a "complete" breakfast, meaning three of the food groups, like dairy, grain and protein.

Here's the good news about not skipping meals: The Girlfriends Diet includes snacks so that you don't go through the day for more than three or four hours without food. Snacks, however, are not mini meals. Keep them in the range of 80 to 100 calories, just enough to keep your metabolism tuned and your appetite under control. Ideally, try to keep your snacks nutritious and protein-oriented, such as an apple with a little peanut butter, a small handful of almonds or an ounce of light cheese.

Lay off the 'no-fat, fill-me-up' store-bought snacks. I can't think of anything worse!"

Manufacturers like to lure you with the no-fat come-on, but what you're getting in many diet processed foods is pure refined carbohydrates. It's like eating a stack of white bread! It's no-fat with plenty of calories.

Snack on the foods people in the Mediterranean eat—nutrient-dense fresh fruit or nuts such as almonds and pistachios. Or carry a healthy snack bar in your purse or briefcase so you're never stuck for something to eat. See our recommended healthy snacks on page 275.

GF Habit No. 6 » *Know your portion sizes.*

Virtually every girlfriend featured in this book had the same thing to say about what they considered to be the most important secret to their successful weight loss: portion control. If you don't know *exactly* how much you're eating, you can't count calories. If you don't count calories, you're not going to lose weight.

To prepare for The Girlfriends Diet, you need to:

* Stock your refrigerator with fruits and vegetables, using the foods featured in Chapter 4 as your guide, and get familiar with their calorie counts

* Get rid of your white rice, pasta and other grains, and replace them with whole wheat products

* Get rid of any sugar-laden products in your pantry

* Invest in measuring cups, measuring spoons and an easy way you can look up calorie counts, like an app on your phone or a book. Also, some people find the precision of a kitchen scale that can measure food in ounces to be very helpful.

Top 10 Girl-Friendly Snacks

Those 100-calorie snack packs are great in a pinch, but if you want to snack for nutrition, reach for a piece of fruit or some crunchy veggies like carrots, celery, broccoli or radishes. You're sure to be in the 80- to 100-calorie range. Or try these girlfriend-tested favorites:

1. A large hard-boiled egg sprinkled with sea salt and paprika: **80** calories

2. Six medium shrimp with ¼ c. cocktail sauce: **84** calories

3. 1 c. raw snap peas and dip made with ¼ c. Greek yogurt with about ½ tsp. each of balsamic vinegar and olive oil: **88** calories

4. Ice pop made with 1 c. each low-fat vanilla yogurt, berries and fruit juice (like pineapple or orange) pureed in a blender and frozen (makes 4 pops): **94** calories each

5. One medium apple, sliced, sprinkled with cinnamon: **95** calories

6. Cherry tomatoes, halved, topped with 2 Tbsp. (1 oz.) goat cheese and sprinkled with fresh pepper or chives: **96** calories

7. ½ whole wheat mini bagel, toasted, topped with a wedge of Laughing Cow Strawberries & Cream cheese spread and a sliced strawberry: **107** calories

8. Toasted baguette slice topped with 1 Tbsp. ricotta cheese, chopped fresh oregano, black pepper and an (optional) anchovy fillet, broiled until melted and drizzled with olive oil: **108** calories (116 calories with anchovy)

9. Veggie burger (such as Boca, Gardenburger or Dr. Praeger's) on an iceberg lettuce "bun" with a little yellow mustard: **100** calories

10. 2 Tbsp. blanched almonds: **105** calories

Using measuring cups and spoons and weighing food is a good way to keep exact control of your calorie intake. Eyeballing is a habit that can get some people into trouble. We proved this when we brought a group of dieters to our Good Housekeeping test kitchens and asked them to "measure" ingredients without using measuring spoons. Instead, we asked them to use their own instincts as their guide. They overestimated on every count, adding from 160 to 180 calories on each individual item.

GF STAY SLIM SECRET

"I don't eat low-fat or fat-free products. Instead, I keep tabs on my portions. Every few weeks I pick one day to measure meals and snacks. It's funny how that half cup of ice cream easily grows to three-quarters of a cup when you're just eyeballing it. Measuring everything every day would be a big hassle, so this reality check is an easier way to help me stay on track."

—*Karen Birong, 44, Minneapolis, MN*

The recipes in this book are important in helping you learn what a portion size should be. However, losing and maintaining weight means you must get familiar with portion size independent of weight-loss recipes. *Measure* a tablespoon of salad dressing and put it in a bowl. That's what it should look like when you sprinkle (don't pour) it on your salad. *Measure* a tablespoon of oil and put it in a pan. That's the amount you need to sauté vegetables. Slice and weigh an ounce of cheese and put it on a plate. Measure out a half cup of pasta and place it on a plate.

To give you a sense of what some typical serving sizes are, here are some visual equivalents you can use if you don't have a scale:

Skip the Diet Soda

Why do you find diet soda on menus in Mediterranean countries? Because visiting Americans ask for it!

Diet cola may be zero calories, but you should not sip it all day long. Tufts University researchers found that women who regularly drink three or more regular or diet colas a week have lower bone-mineral density than those who sip less, because the caffeine and phosphoric acid in soda may interfere with calcium absorption and bone strength.

* Fish, poultry, meat—3 ounces—a smartphone

* Cheese—1 ounce—four dice

* Salad dressing—1 tablespoons—half a shot glass

* Grains, pasta and rice—½ cup—a tennis ball

* Nuts—a quarter cup—an egg

GF Habit No. 7 » *Eat most of your calories before 3 P.M.*

It's a Mediterranean custom to eat the largest meal of the day at lunch—a tactic that's been proven to help make the weight come off faster. Garaulet has found this to be consistent in the thousands of people she has helped lose weight. In 2013, she published a study involving 420 patients in her weight-loss clinic who were divided into two groups: early eaters (those who had their main meal before 3 P.M.) and late eaters (those who had their main meal after 3 P.M.). "Late eaters lost less weight and displayed a slower weight-loss rate during the 20 weeks of treatment, even though other factors were essentially the same—calorie intake and expenditure, appetite hormones and even sleep duration," the study found.

While eating a leisurely lunch as the main meal isn't the lifestyle of the typical American woman, you can diet Mediterranean-style by eating most of your calories before 3 P.M. This means that you want to make sure to eat breakfast, lunch and any snacks by 3 P.M. Previous studies indicate that people who eat more of their daily calories at night have a higher propensity to put on weight and less ability to lose it. It also helps explain why studies have found that shift workers are more prone to obesity than day workers, even if their caloric input and output are the same. Research also indicates that late eaters are more likely to eat poorer-quality breakfasts or to skip the meal altogether.

"These results emphasize that timing of food intake may play a significant role in weight regulation," says Garaulet. She believes a lot of it has to do with our internal clock—what scientists call circadian rhythms. Research shows that the circadian clock influences how the body stores and mobilizes fat. Also, eating the majority of your calories early may help improve the way your body uses insulin, which improves digestion speed.

"Overweight people often have to reprogram their idea of 'enough.' To figure out portions, use your eyes, not your stomach. A serving of nuts, for example, is two tablespoons."
—*Alice Bosley,* Good Housekeeping *reader, Clarkston, MI*

GF Habit No. 8 » *Don't put foods off-limits; put limits on certain foods.*

When we asked a group of girlfriends what treat they could never live without, nearly half—47%—said it was a chocolate pick-me-up. Next came ice cream at 29%, Friday-night pizza at 16% and chips with lunch at 8%. Really, anyone surprised?!

This is why no food is off-limits on The Girlfriends Diet. *Say that again?* the skeptic in you asks. No need—you heard us right. On The Girlfriends Diet you don't have to give up your favorite foods.

But, the skeptic within persists, *eating my favorite foods is the reason I gained weight in the first place!* Well, yes, but more likely the truth is this: The real reason you ended up with a real weight problem is *because* you tried to fight it by abandoning the foods you love.

There's a scientific explanation why following a diet that denies you certain foods doesn't work. Dieters who restrict themselves too much—who give up the pizza and French bread they love, or give up an entire food category such as carbohydrates—start yearning for what they are denying themselves in just a matter of *days*.

It's a proven fact, borne out by mountains of research and anecdotal evidence, including the work conducted by obesity expert Janet Polivy, Ph.D., and her colleagues at the University of Toronto. Even anticipated deprivation—*I'm going for it big-time tonight because the diet starts tomorrow*—can trigger the mother of all binges. There's even a name for it: Last Supper Effect.

"It's all about survival. You can't go without eating. It's like trying to hold your breath indefinitely underwater," says America's most trusted doctor, Mehmet Oz, M.D., host of *The Dr. Oz Show* and a cardiac surgeon at New York-Presbyterian Hospital/Columbia University Medical Center in New York City. "So your body has a very concrete set of systems that reinforces the need for you to eat."

It's the reason you shouldn't skip meals—and the reason you don't have to give up your favorite treats. The problem with deprivation is "you violate the biology of blubber," says Dr. Oz. When you're trying to lose weight, your body is rarely up for it. Your brain doesn't interpret "diet" the way you want it to—as a way of slimming down so you can slip into a pencil skirt. After you lose those first few pounds with your first few days of this-time-I'm-determined willpower, your brain sends a panicked alert to your body, *I want my chips! I gotta have them!*

So have your chips. Just count out the number so you know the exact amount of calories and include them in your tally for your meal. And don't have chips every day. Consider them an occasional treat. It's likely that as you eat them less often, you'll want them less. Studies show that when we start nurturing ourselves with nutritious

Dear GF,

At about 100 calories an ounce—some types of cheese are a little more or a little less—we can see why having a "cheese-tooth" can trip you up. The trap you're setting for yourself is trying to avoid it—IMPOSSIBLE! What you need to do is feed your craving with some lighter options that are low in calories but don't taste like it. Try these the next time a slice of Brie is calling your name:

* *Light string cheese* is just like the real thing—and it's fun to pull apart. Each stick has only about 50 or 60 calories. Rip it into shreds for the cheese topping on your mini personal veggie pizza.
* *Laughing Cow Light* wedges at 35 calories a pop can't be beat for spreadable cheese. Try one on a 100-calorie bagel in place of cream cheese, on high-fiber crackers, or on apple and pear slices.
* *Mini Babybel* cheese rounds are terrific, if hard cheese is your thing. At 50 calories for the light variety and 60 to 80 calories for the regular version, they just can't be outdone.
* *Cabot Vermont Serious Snacking reduced fat cheese bars* really are for serious cheese freaks. The flavors—from zesty to super-spicy—are awesome. We love the pepper jack! And they're just 50 calories or fewer each.

foods, our dependency on less nutritious, fattening foods starts to dissipate. The change can be so simple—and produce remarkable results. Researchers in Quebec proved this when they helped 77 healthy women with a sweet tooth give up sweets by having them eat more legumes, nuts and seeds in place of their usual treats. They underwent dietary counseling to help them through the 12-week test stage. Their efforts paid off big in terms of "significant decreases in body weight and waist circumference" during the three-month study.

So, how do you adopt diet plan designed to change your eating habits while still allowing for your favorite foods? By learning new habits that will help make sticking to the diet a no-brainer. Plus, your new routines will help ensure that you'll continue to keep up the good work and maintain your new weight after you reach your weight-loss goal, so all your efforts will not have been for naught.

That's why you should think of The Girlfriends Diet as a diet of addition, not subtraction. By concentrating on all the good foods you should eat, your mind will have little time to get fixated on what you shouldn't eat. Tell yourself each day that planning your daily meals and snacks around what's best for your body means you'll be reaching for fruits and vegetables, which are naturally low in calories and high in nutrients, as well as protein, at every meal. You'll see—and will probably be surprised—that you won't get between-

⊱ Fast-Food Cravings—Gone! ⊰

Want to kick the fast-food habit? No problem. Just start eating healthier, and your desire for not-so-healthy food will start to disappear.

Canadian researchers put this assumption to the test by recruiting 71 young and middle-aged women to try to eat better by taking up a Mediterranean diet. The women were given the parameters of the diet—lots of fruits and veggies, good grains, minimal red meat, etc.—and sent on their way for a 12-week tryout. Their only instructions: Record what you eat each day. Words like "weight loss" and "fast food" were not part of the lecture.

As the women adjusted more and more to eating the Mediterranean way, their interest in fast food declined accordingly. In fact, the women who adhered the most to the healthier diet showed the least interest in fast food. To top it off, they lost a "significant" amount of weight.

The researchers' bottom line: The cure for eating unhealthy foods is to start eating and enjoying healthy foods.

meal hunger like you used to because you'll be eating enough calories throughout the day to put your body's starvation meter on snooze. That's why it's important that you never go below 1,200 calories a day. When you eat fat, protein and fiber at each meal, you'll feel fuller longer and your desire for that food you think you can't do without will gradually go away. But should temptation get

AMASING! MAKEOVER!
Karen Birong
"I lost 195 pounds—and became a personal trainer!"

I GREW UP WITH a "clean your plate" mentality and was inactive as a child. I became heavier as I got older, but it never really bothered me. My parents did a great job encouraging my self-esteem, and I didn't think of my weight as an obstacle. A friend once told me that my personality was bigger than my size!

When I turned 40 in May 2009, I was over 300 pounds, always tired and could barely reach down to put on my socks. I also started taking high blood pressure medication. My husband was helping out his ailing parents, and I

thought: *I cannot be the next person he has to take care of—we are supposed to be a team.* I vowed to make changes.

I decided to revamp my eating habits in the new year. So in January 2010, I cut my daily calories from around 4,000 to 1,800—I replaced burgers and fries with lean pork chops and green beans, swapped butter for Greek yogurt and gave up sugary pop cold turkey. I also tracked what I ate in a food journal. My mantra: *If I bite it, I write it.* I kept protein shakes in the fridge at all times. They were a filling meal-replacement option

for busy days or when I didn't feel like cooking. After four weeks, I had lost 20 pounds. That's when I decided to go to the gym—the one I had belonged to for over a year and only went to *once*. I got on the treadmill and could only do 10 minutes. It was deflating. So, I signed an 18-month contract for a twice-a-week personal trainer to learn how to do weights and cardio.

The person who evaluated me asked if I cared if she paired me up with a guy personal trainer. Cared? Of course I cared! I was nervous and scared, the best of you and you reach for a handful of potato chips, or a chocolate chip cookie, know that it's OK. "You don't have to have a lot of it," says Dr. Oz. "A small chocolate chip cookie won't kill you." The difference between the you of the past and the you of the future is that you're going to learn to be aware of food in ways that prevent you from caving in and eating the whole bag of cookies or chips, the

but I said OK anyway. As it turned out, D.K. came to be the missing piece that helped me achieve my 195-pound weight-loss success. At first, I didn't think he thought I could do it, and every day after I left the gym, I cried. But after one week, I lost five pounds, and the second week, I lost another five pounds. That's when he said, "I think we should take some measurements." He always believed I could do it—he and my skinny husband.

Today, I am a new person. I never lost my self-esteem, which is good. I've lost 195 pounds and I am off all my meds. I always eat healthy—it's just the kind of food I like now—and I go to the gym five or six times a week.

"It's amazing what a group environment can do to keep people motivated."

But twice a week D.K. and I still work out together. We have a bond that can't be broken. Last spring, I got my personal trainer license, and D.K. and I teamed up to run a weight-loss challenge at the gym. I do the classroom portion

in my home and then we all go over to the gym for the boot camp, which D.K. leads. It's amazing what a group environment can do to keep people motivated. I've found that people do really well when they get that kind of support!

D.K. was the key factor in my weight loss, and he's now like a member of our family. And with my renewed health, I now look forward to an adventurous future with my husband.

whole carton of ice cream or the whole plate of nachos. You'll be eating fewer processed foods, which are sneaky sources of sugar, which means you'll naturally be dialing down your sweet tooth. Pretty soon, sweet things will taste too sweet, so you'll want less of them.

Cravings become fewer and farther between when you don't give in to them. However, we all get cravings from time to time. We wouldn't be human otherwise. Heck, even Dr. Oz gets cravings. "I go crazy over chocolate-covered nuts," he says. "I just love the combination—the way they taste in my mouth, the texture, the smell. It's fantastic." But he has a simple trick that makes him resist going whole hog. "I take one handful, never more than that, and then I drink a big glass of water. You'll see. The water will wash the taste from your mouth. The taste buds have already been satisfied, and the craving will stop. Then just step away."

GF Habit No. 9 » When the going gets tough, enlist the 80/20 rule

So you ate the whole thing? Well, so what. The diet's not over. Even if it looks like you've blown your diet royally by eating everything you could poke your fork into at the buffet table, just swallow your

⊰ Think Twice About Sugar ⊱

Okay, when we say nothing is off-limits, that includes sugar. But when the temptation is getting to you, ask yourself, *Just how badly do I want that piece of cake?*

We've been hearing it since we were kids: *Sugar is empty calories*—no nutritional value. But there is an even more important reason why we should avoid it as much as possible. Researchers say sugar is closely related to the current U.S. obesity and diabetes epidemics.

Instead, feed your sugar craving with a piece of fruit.

guilt, forgive yourself and get back on board immediately. You didn't do any permanent damage, research conducted by the National Institutes of Health (NIH) reveals. NIH researchers created a model that simulated a person's food intake and found that even if your weight fluctuates by 600 calories a day, you still won't gain or lose more than three pounds over a decade.

The Girlfriends Diet is not about perfection, so there's no need to aim for it. The only way for you to truly stick to a healthy diet and take off excess weight *permanently* is to realize you can't be a saint about what you eat 24/7. When you catch yourself going off track, implement the 80/20 rule in order to counter the "What-the-Hell Effect." You know how it goes: You have your usual oatmeal and a banana for breakfast and get a healthy takeout salad for lunch. But the rest of the office had a different idea and brought in pizza—and the smell is driving you nuts. You resist and resist until your resistance says, *One sliver of a slice can't hurt.* Only the sliver turns into the whole slice and then you reach for a second. That's when the What-the-Hell Effect sets in, as in *What the hell—now that I've blown my diet, I might as well dig in and enjoy what I can't have for the rest of the day and get back to eating healthy tomorrow.* You stop at KFC on your way home, and later on, you treat yourself to some ice cream before you go to bed.

However, you don't want to turn a 600-calorie mistake into a 6,000-calorie mistake. This *will* get you in trouble. That's like taking a wrong turn and continuing on instead of turning around and getting back on the right track again. You'll never get to where you want to be. If you overeat at one meal, don't rationalize that today's ruined and then continue to eat everything in sight, vowing you'll get back on it tomorrow. Instead, once you've acknowledged your indulgence, get up from the table or, as Dr. Oz suggests (see page 84), have a glass of water to dampen the craving, and then move on.

Enlisting the 80/20 plan will also put the brakes on this type of behavior, says Alice Domar, Ph.D., executive director of the Domar Center for Mind/Body Health, and the author of six books. "Letting yourself indulge in moderation is key," Domar says. Consider that piece of pizza (or two) the 20%—your so-called slipup, or indulgence, for the day—and maintain your 80% healthy eating throughout the rest of the day. By consuming healthy fare most of the time and allowing yourself the occasional treat, you can counter the What-the-Hell Effect.

GF Habit No. 10 » *Get more active and change your mind-set about food*

The trifecta of successful weight loss is: a healthy diet, daily activity and appropriate behavior practices about and around food. It's like that with *any* weight-loss program. Though research shows that exercise alone does not lead to weight loss—or at least makes it very difficult—exercise *does* make calorie restriction work better and, often, even faster. It also builds muscle, which boosts metabolism. "Data have demonstrated that even when exercise energy expenditure is high, a healthy diet is still required for weight loss to occur in many people," report researchers from the University of Leeds in the United Kingdom. Research conducted in Spain shows that a low-calorie Mediterranean-style diet coupled with exercise is the ideal combo because it is scientifically proven to improve quality of life, both physically and mentally. You'll find the Girlfriends approach to getting active in Chapter 7.

Adjusting your behavior around food, however, is the key to making all your hard effort pay off for the long haul. Theoretically, losing weight through diet should be easy, since it consists of producing an energy deficit in which energy intake is less than energy expenditure, note experts. However, in the course of attempting to lose weight, most people encounter a number of obstacles and barriers—the habits they've adopted over a lifetime that caused the weight gain in the first place. "It is especially difficult to instill correct eating habits in modern-day society, where it is so easy to obtain tasty, high-calorie food and where any celebration is an excuse for overeating," says Garaulet. She's found that practicing behavior therapy by training the brain to change its mind-set about food helps her weight-loss clients.

"Behavior therapy is based on the classic principles of 'conditioning,' which indicate that eating is frequently associated with environmental events and cues linked to eating," says Garaulet. The underlying principle is that our thoughts directly affect our emotions and, as a consequence, our actions. In other words, people who struggle with weight loss eat for reasons other than hunger. Our mind is the reason we overeat, why we gain weight and why we lose it only to gain it back again. Without correcting these behaviors, we are doomed to repeat the mistakes of the past that lead to weight gain. The mind is so key to making new habits stick and to putting bad habits behind you, we've devoted Chapter 5 to it entirely.

Banning Gluten Is Not a Weight-Loss Secret

Gluten, a protein found in wheat, rye and barley that is getting a lot of attention these days, has nothing to do with gaining weight. In fact, if you switch from regular bread, pasta, rice, crackers and cookies to gluten-free products, you might end up adding on pounds.

Packaged foods in "the gluten-free varieties are often higher in sugar, fat and calories than regular versions," says Rachel Begun, M.S., R.D., spokesperson for the Academy of Nutrition and Dietetics. If you're wondering why that girlfriend who gave up gluten looks slimmer, it's probably because she cut back on high-calorie packaged foods like muffins, cakes and crackers—that's a smart move for anyone. If you do likewise, and replace these products with unprocessed, naturally gluten-free foods like girl-friendly fruits, vegetables, meats, low-fat dairy, nuts and beans, you will lose weight, too. "But that's because you're eating an overall healthier diet, not because you eliminated gluten," says Begun.

The only people who need to avoid gluten are those who experience symptoms when they eat it. See your doctor if you have bloating or abdominal pain (especially after eating) and suspect you might have Celiac disease—a chronic, often debilitating, condition in which gluten damages the lining of the small intestines so your body can't absorb crucial nutrients from food. No matter what, if you decide to go gluten-free, visit your doctor first.

GF Action Plan

ADJUST AND KEEP RECORDING YOUR CALORIES. Now that you know how many calories you should be consuming, start your diet! And remember to record not only what you're eating, but also any changes you feel physically and emotionally so you can share them with your Girlfriends Diet Club pals.

ADOPT YOUR NEW STYLE OF EATING. Here's a quick list of Mediterranean versus non-Mediterranean foods. Keep this with you when you go grocery shopping and are planning menus as a quick reference guide.

Mediterranean Foods	Non-Mediterranean Foods
Cereals	Butter and butter substitutes
Dairy (low-fat)	Fast food
Fish	Processed meats and other foods
Fruits	Red meat
Grains	Soft drinks
Legumes	Sugar
Nuts	
Olive oil	
Potatoes	
Vegetables	
Wine	

START SLOWLY. If your current pattern of eating doesn't include lots of fruits and vegetables and other plant-based foods, you might want to ease into the diet gradually. Each day add more and more of these foods to your plate. If you slip up at one meal, pick up at the next.

PRACTICE THE 10 GF HABITS. Review them daily and plan your eating accordingly. They're meant to be, well, habit-forming.

The Girlfriends Diet Food Basket

WHAT EXACTLY *IS* MEDITERRANEAN-STYLE food anyway? Granted, just the image of the Mediterranean—warm days, a deep blue sea, perpetual sunshine—conjures up eating that is both luscious and exotic, something you might experience in a restaurant or on a trip, but not necessarily something easy enough to take up as an everyday lifestyle at home. The reality: luscious, yes, but exotic, not so much. Rather, it is practical. Simple, even. And it is *easy* to adopt. Anyone born in the regions surrounding the Mediterranean will tell you that the best food is found in the home, not the restaurant!

This is one of the reasons why a Mediterranean-style approach got two thumbs up as the eating style of choice on The Girlfriends Diet. That and the fact that it's just so darn healthy and tasty—the kinds of foods that appeal to women. You can't argue with the science that shows that eating in the style of some of the healthiest and most robust people in the world is the way to go. Research has shown that people who adhere the most to a Mediterranean diet weigh less and have a lower rate of heart disease, cancer, depression and neurological diseases. It all comes from eating from the Mediterranean food basket—fruits, vegetables, grains and other natural choices that also happen to be the foods with the widest variety and highest content of beneficial health-bestowing compounds. These nutrients include carotenes; lycopene; lutein; the antioxidant nutrient selenium; vitamins A, D, E and folate; a variety of flavonoids; omega-3 fatty acids; monounsaturated and polyunsaturated fats; and lots of soluble and unsoluble fiber. Scientists believe these nutrients found in the foods common to the Mediterranean work synergistically in their own special way to protect us against a variety of chronic conditions. Unlike American-style eating, these foods don't show up as an afterthought on the dining plate—a side to a slab of meat. Rather, they get star billing. Meat is nice, but just a little will do, thank you!

So how do you follow suit, planning fruits and vegetables to take up half of your plate, with extra room for grains and legumes? By selecting from this list of foods we call the Girl-Friendly 42. These are all nutrient-dense foods that are commonly eaten in the Mediterranean and believed to be among the healthiest in the world. These are the foods from which you can pick and choose every day to include in your eating plan—and they're readily available in the average supermarket.

It's why we say it is a diet of *addition*, not subtraction. On The Girlfriends Diet, when you wake up in the morning, you'll be thinking about all the wonderful foods you'll *want* to eat—deliciousness you can look forward to throughout the day. Concentrate on eating the Mediterranean's best of the best—foods, by the way, that are nutritious and calorie-considerate—and you won't be lamenting the foods that have helped put you at the weight you are today. It's *the*

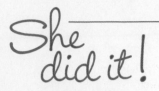

She did it!

TALAYA ROOKS
AGE **44**
LOST **13 POUNDS!**

HERE'S HOW: "With four kids, a full-time job and a husband who travels on business quite a bit, it's hard to always eat right and maintain a consistent exercise routine. I wasn't overweight, but I wanted to feel like my old self. I'm always encouraging my kids to play sports. Now it's like, 'Here's Mommy's challenge'—so they can see me as a role model.

"I had 10 pounds to lose, so I thought it would be easy, but the weight did not come off quickly at first. I stuck it out though, healthy eating and workouts, and soon my clothes started fitting better. Instead of having dessert, like I used to, now I just have a piece of fruit. Eventually the weight came off—I surpassed my goal and lost 13 pounds. I'm fitting into clothes I haven't worn in 20 years."

diet that gives you your best chance to achieve what's most important to your health—the ability to attain and maintain your perfect weight and resist chronic and debilitating health issues.

Remember, it's not that you can never, never, ever have chocolate fudge cheesecake or mac with double cheese again. (OK, maybe you *should* skip the double and go easy on the sugar.) You just need to learn how to eat them *responsibly*—and we'll get to that in Chapter 5.

Now, here's the deal. Don't think of this list as "diet" food; think of it as your blueprint for a delicious and healthier lifestyle. Eat healthy, and weight loss will follow if you use this formula: Select *at least* five vegetables and three fruits a day, plus a whole grain at each meal, to add to the fish, poultry, meat or other protein you choose. Remember, the ratio is one-half fruits and vegetables; one-quarter grains or cereals; and one-quarter protein, including plant protein such as beans, chickpeas or nuts. Also, make sure your plate is colorful—reds, blues and especially greens. Eat like this every day, and your body will start to pay you back—inside and out. You'll gradually lose excess pounds, feel a lift in your energy levels, and garner some or all of the many health benefits that have made the world's top experts in food and nutrition declare the Mediterranean diet the healthiest in the world and your best chance of attaining permanent weight loss.

To help you make your choices, we searched the scientific literature to find out the healthful reasons *why* you should eat these foods. We also suggest *how* you can eat them, the best time to buy them and their nutritive value. We even offer some inside secrets. So read up, and dig in.

APPLES

Why you should eat them » An apple a day...well, you know. Apples contain an amazing array of polyphenols, including quercitin, a compound that protects brain cells from tissue-damaging free radicals. And there's more: A study at Florida State University found that women who ate 2.6 ounces of dried apples (roughly equal to one fresh apple) every day for a year saw their bad cholesterol drop by a considerable 23%. As for weight loss, researchers at Penn State found that eating an apple 15 minutes before lunch can cut 200 calories out of your daily diet.

How you can eat them » Toss a chopped McIntosh into a spinach salad with walnuts and some low-fat feta cheese, or thinly slice a Granny Smith on a turkey sandwich for a sweet and tart crunch.

Best time to buy » Most are at their peak from early fall through the end of October. Get the family in on good eating choices by taking the kids to a local orchard to pick their own.

Insider tip » That bruising you see when you drop an apple and the browning that occurs after cutting into one are signs of escaping polyphenols. So when you're eating a raw apple, have the peel, too, which houses a lot of the nutrients.

Nutritional tally » One medium apple comes in at 95 calories and delivers 20% of your daily fiber needs, making it one of the best single sources of dietary fiber. An apple a day is right-on advice.

The Girl-Friendly Pantry

Keep these girl-friendly convenience foods and staples at the ready to have on hand when cooking from The Girlfriends Diet Food Basket:

* A variety of dried and canned beans
* A variety of nuts such as almonds, walnuts and pistachios
* Brown rice, including frozen brown rice
* Whole-grain cereals, pastas and crackers
* Canned white albacore tuna and salmon
* Frozen vegetables
* Herbs and spices
* Olive oil and canola oil
* Artichoke hearts
* Low-sodium, low-fat chicken and vegetable broths
* A jar of chopped garlic
* Canned tomato products

ARTICHOKES

Why you should eat them » The health benefits of artichokes come from the copious amounts of heart-protecting phenolic compounds they contain, which can help bring down total cholesterol and dangerous LDL cholesterol, and help keep blood sugar under control.

How you can eat them » 'Chokes look medieval (all those thorns), but they're surprisingly simple to prepare. Choose bulbs with tightly closed leaves, then wash, trim the stem and boil until the leaves peel away easily, about 45 min. Forget the butter and serve with this tangy sauce: ¼ c. reduced-fat mayo; ¼ c. Greek yogurt; juice from 1 lemon; and 2 cloves of garlic, minced. Also tasty: Toss thawed frozen artichoke hearts into salads or pasta.

Best time to buy » Artichokes' peak season is the spring, but they are harvested year-round in California, where most artichokes in U.S. markets come from.

Insider tip » If fiddling with artichoke leaves is too much for you, go for canned. The healthy compounds can be found even in commercially canned artichoke hearts.

Nutritional tally » A whole artichoke has only 76 calories but an astounding nine grams of fiber, more than a third of what you need in a day.

ASPARAGUS

Why you should eat it » The quintessential spring veggie offers a unique combination of anti-inflammatory nutrients and a wide variety of antioxidants, including beta-carotene and vitamins C and E—a combo that puts asparagus among the best risk reducers for common chronic health problems.

How you can eat it » To prep, snap off the ends and discard, then blanch and toss into salads, add to a stir-fry or frittata; or roll in a little olive oil, sprinkle with shredded Pecorino Romano and roast in

The GF Hangover Helper

Never mind coffee or the hair of the dog. When a state of misery originates from one too many cocktails the night before, steam up some asparagus. According to a *Journal of Food Science* report, it's chock-full of special amino acids (asparagin, aspartic acid) that mop up aldehydes—main hangover culprits. For faster relief, blend with water and drink as a juice.

a 400°F oven for 10 to 15 min. until the cheese is nicely melted.

Best time to buy » Asparagus is at its absolute best during its spring harvesting season. It is on the Environmental Working Group's "clean 15" list of produce least likely to be contaminated by pesticides so there's no need to buy organic.

Insider tip » To pick a good bunch, hold it up to your ear, then gently squeeze and twist. If the stalks squeak when rubbed against each other, then they're fresh.

Nutritional tally » A dieter's dream: A miniscule 40 calories, a rich three grams of fiber, and a noteworthy five grams of protein per cup. One cup also contains an impressive 70% of your daily minimum requirement for vitamins D and K.

AVOCADOS

Why you should eat them » Once vilified as a weight-loss no-no for its high fat content—85%!—the avocado is now considered a nutritional superhero because most of that fat is monounsaturated, the kind that is a savior to the heart. The green flesh is a sign that it oozes with another heart-healthy antioxidant: beta-carotene. We can also put the "but it's fattening" controversy to rest. When researchers put a group of women on a low-fat, nutrient-dense diet that included two daily servings of avocado as part of a salad or salsa, no one gained weight and half of the women actually lost weight.

How you can eat them » In their natural state, as heat starts to dissipate their ample supply of nutrients. Sliced or mashed, they are an ingenious swap for butter, cream cheese or mayo on your morning toast or lunchtime sandwich. Adding sliced or chopped avocado increases the beta-carotene in the greens of an otherwise avocado-free salad. Mix chopped avocado with onions, tomatoes, lime juice, cumin and cilantro for a different twist on guacamole. Use it as a spread, instead of mayo, on sandwiches and in chicken salad.

Best time to buy » Any time. Different types of avocado are in peak season at different times of the year.

Insider tip » Most of the carotenoids in an avocado are found in the deep-green flesh right under the skin. To keep them intact, peel with your hands as you would a banana.

Nutritional tally » They're not as high in calories as you might think: Half a medium-size avocado contains about 110 calories, 10 grams of fiber and 13 grams of good-for-you monounsaturated fat—nearly three-quarters of its fat content.

WHAT THE **FOOD** EXPERTS SAY

"Every dietitian I know agrees that avocados are a must-eat food. They are a great source of healthy fats, which help fill you up so you'll be less likely to want a snack later. Plus, they taste really decadent."
—*Carolyn Brown, R.D. at Foodtrainers, New York City*

BANANAS

Why you should eat them » Bananas offer us riches in potassium, an essential mineral for maintaining normal blood pressure and a healthy heart.

How you can eat them » Slice them over hot oatmeal and cold cereal. Peel, cut in half, insert a popsicle stick in the cut end, dip the tip in a little melted dark chocolate and freeze for a snack or dessert.

Best time to buy » Bananas grow in warm climates all year round, making them a prime buy any time of the year.

Insider tip » Eat a banana as a snack when you hit an afternoon slump. Research shows that bananas provide more carbohydrates and energizing nutrients like potassium than sports drinks do.

Nutritional tally » Some shun them for being "too caloric," but, hey, they're still a fruit and have virtually no fat. One medium banana delivers about 100 calories, three grams of fiber, 17% of our minimum daily requirement of vitamin C and a whopping 467 milligrams of potassium.

BEANS

Why you should eat them » They are one of the healthiest sources of vegetable protein you can find. And they're super-nutritious, containing a collection of phytonutrients and other bioactive compounds, including cholesterol-lowering soluble fiber, which helps reduce the risk of obesity, heart disease, cancer and diabetes. Putting beans in your diet also contributes to weight loss. When a bean-based low-calorie diet was measured against a low-calorie diet containing no beans, researchers found that four servings of beans a week was responsible for reducing weight, blood pressure, cholesterol and chronic inflammation in obese people.

How you can eat them » We aren't suggesting that you live on beans alone, but if you wanted to, you could, without ever getting bored. There are at least 70 varieties of beans, plus other legumes such as lentils, chickpeas and peas, to choose from and an infinite number of ways to make them—in soups, salads and casseroles.

Best way to buy » If time allows, opt for dried beans over canned. Some research suggests that some nutritional value in canned beans is lost through processing. When using canned beans, rinse under cold water first to get rid of excess salt.

Insider tip » One study found that when people included chickpeas in their diets, they reached for fewer processed high-fat snack foods. Bring on the hummus!

The Super Swap: Sugar to Honey

Skip the refined white stuff and swirl a teaspoon or two of antioxidant-laced "liquid gold" into your oatmeal, tea or even coffee. The switch could affect hunger hormones in slimming ways, according to a University of Wyoming study. Compared with sugar, honey delayed the rise of ghrelin, a hormone that drives us to eat, and boosted levels of the feel-full appetite peptide (a protein-like substance) called PYY. *Suh-weet!*

Honey does add calories though—22 per teaspoon—so drizzle, don't drench.

Nutritional tally » It depends on the beans, but most contain around 100 filling calories per half cup, with no fat and about eight grams of protein. Black beans are considered to be nutritionally superior to other beans.

BEETS

Why you should eat them » Beets' claim to nutritional fame is their unusual mix of antioxidants—hence their bleeding-red color—and for their status as a rare source of betalains, which makes them a great detox agent.

How you can eat them » For no-mess prep, wrap beets in foil and roast at 425°F for 45 min. Let cool, then use a paper towel to slide the skins off. Cut them into chunks, add toothpicks and dip them into low-calorie salad dressing for a snack. Long cooking tends to dissipate betalains, so keep steaming time under 15 min. and roasting time under 1 hr.

Best time to buy » Beets are planted in the spring and harvested in the fall. Choose small bulbs, as they're more tender.

Insider tip » When buying fresh beets, don't throw out the leaves. They are incredibly nutritious in their own right, including being a rich source of beta-carotene. Prepare them as you would spinach.

Nutritional tally » 58 calories, four grams of fiber and a third of your daily folate needs per cup.

BELL PEPPERS

Why you should eat them » Talk about filling your plate with a rainbow of colors—you can do it just with bell peppers! The vibrant palette of bells—red, green, yellow, orange and even purple, brown and black—are an advertisement that they are rich in disease-fighting carotenoids and phenolic compounds that protect against the degenerative diseases of aging.

How you can eat them » Roast peppers on the grill until charred and sweet, and add to sandwiches or puree into pasta sauce. Blend together red bells, chickpeas and tahini to make homemade hummus.

Best time to buy » Bells are available in marketplaces all year round, but you'll find taste at its peak and prices the lowest during summer. Scout for locally grown bells in farmers' markets.

Insider tip » Be partial to the red ones. They are simply riper versions of the green ones, and because they spend more time in the sun while on the plant, they develop more nutrients and fiber. Just half a medium red bell pepper offers up your day's supply of skin-repairing vitamin A and more than your day's supply of immunity-boosting vitamin C.

Nutritional tally » One bell pepper provides 50% more vitamin C than what's found in an orange, delivering 290% of our minimum daily need. It also contains 105% of the minimum daily requirement for vitamin A. To make it even better, all this nutrition comes with a minimum of calories—just 30 to 40 calories in one cup.

BERRIES

Why you should eat them » Good things *do* come in small packages. Be they blue, black, or red—*all* berries are nutritional powerhouses, packed with health-giving antioxidants: Think cancer fighter, heart helper, brain booster. The tiny blueberry gets the most kudos for giving you more nutrients per bite than any other fruit. In fact, one study found that the polyphenols in blueberries prolonged a spike in metabolism after people exercised.

How you can eat them » Pop 'em plain or toss them into your oatmeal or yogurt. Make them into a sauce atop poultry or fish. For a colorful Mediterranean-style salsa, toss 1 c. blueberries with ½ diced avocado, ¼ c. diced red onion, 1 Tbsp. minced and seeded jalapeño, 2 Tbsp. olive oil and the juice of 1 lime.

Best time to buy » Summertime is berry season, but you will get just as much nutrition (and save yourself money) by picking them out of the freezer section of your supermarket.

Insider tip » Berries are among the most pesticide-laden produce items, according to the Environmental Working Group, so go organic if you can—and wash them well if you can't.

Nutritional tally » A cup of berries contains 80 calories or fewer and about as much fiber as a serving of brown rice. But it's their special antioxidants that make for nutritional magic.

WHAT THE FOOD EXPERTS SAY

"A bowl of berries is what most nutritionists have when they're craving something sweet. We favor super-dark berries, like blueberries and blackberries, because they have the highest doses of powerful antioxidants."

—*Keri Glassman, New York City dietitian and author of* The New You and Improved Diet

BROCCOLI

Why you should eat it » It is the hardest-working member of the cancer-fighting cruciferous family (cabbage, brussels sprouts, cauliflower) and the only known vegetable that contains a special trio of important compounds called glucosinates that go after carcinogens full-throttle. Broccoli also contains at least 10 other compounds with well-known cancer-fighting action, including beta-carotene, vitamin C, lutein and quercitin.

How you can eat it » Here's the catch: You mustn't overheat broccoli, or else the enzyme that activates its cancer-fighting agents gets destroyed. Best: Eat it raw or steam it. Steaming actually enhances broccoli's tumor-scavenging agents.

Best way to buy » Look for broccoli with tight clusters that are uniform in color with no yellowing. It can be either dark green, sage or purple-green, depending on the variety.

Insider tip » Buy broccoli whole, not in florets, and don't cut it until you are ready to use. Cutting into it starts to destroy its ample vitamin C content.

Nutritional tally » One cup of steamed broccoli offers 135% of your minimum daily requirement for vitamin C. It's also a rare rich source of folic acid, and it possesses more flavonols than any other vegetable. All that nutrition is bundled in just 54 calories with five grams of fiber.

BROWN RICE

Why you should eat it » Health experts want all of us to make the switch from white rice to brown rice, because the white stuff is high on the glycemic index, making it a chief contributor to the rapid rise in insulin that contributes to weight gain and sharply increases the risk of diabetes. By just swapping out white rice for brown rice, you could reduce your chances of developing type 2 diabetes by 16%, according to research from the Harvard School of Public Health. Type 2 diabetes has nearly doubled among women in the past three decades.

How you can eat it » In all the same ways you eat white rice! Make a super-nutritious pilaf by sautéing green and red bell peppers, diced onions, shredded carrots and broccoli florets in olive oil and stirring it all into the rice. Place a few slices of baked chicken breast on top, and you've got a complete meal.

Best kind to buy » Look for *germinated* brown rice, the "sticky

---

GF WANTS TO KNOW

I'm willing to confess: I hate vegetables. Practically the only ones I eat are carrots and celery. Sometimes I'll eat the tomatoes and lettuce in a sandwich, but salads themselves turn me off. Honestly, it's not that I haven't tried. Is there anything you can do to make a convert out of me?

—Veggies Aren't Me, 32, Brooklyn, NY

Dear GF,

You need help, girlfriend! Vegetables are the core of a Mediterranean-style diet, and they're key to weight loss because they are low in calories and contain plenty of fiber to fill you up—and make you feel satisfied. Our guess is that you've been trying vegetables that are just too boring. The trick is to get creative.

To start, you don't have to eat them as a stand-alone. You can combine them in other foods. For example, add a box of thawed and drained spinach to ground turkey when making burgers or meat loaf. Or, stir veggies like grated carrots or zucchini or broccoli into your pasta sauce.

You should also try roasting vegetables. That really brings out the flavor and makes them much more interesting than a cup of steamed—boring!—veggies sitting on your plate. Ideal roasters: asparagus, brussels sprouts, cauliflower, grape tomatoes, mushrooms, zucchini, winter squash and eggplant. Just cut them into pieces, mist with olive oil spray and roast at 400°F until soft and brown. The high heat gives produce a delicious, nutty flavor that we're betting will make a convert out of you. And here's a **bonus tip:** Drink a glass of V8 juice. Eight ounces is only 50 calories, and it counts as two servings of vegetables!

rice" used to make sushi. It has more nutrients than regular brown rice and is five times more nutritious than white rice. It's also more flavorful than regular brown rice and is easier to cook.

Insider tip » One study found that you can keep white rice from causing an insulin surge by mixing it with a low-glycemic food, such as beans. However, it's still lacking in nutrition.

Nutritional tally » Per ½ cup, brown rice has 108 calories, zero fat and five grams of protein. And the white stuff? Well, so many nutrients are stripped out during the milling process that converts brown rice to white that the federal government mandates that it be enriched with vitamins B1 and B3 and iron.

CABBAGE

Why you should eat it » It deserves plate time much more often than on Saint Patty's Day. Cabbage is a star cancer fighter, owing to its mother lode of glucosinates, which are also what makes cabbage a tad stinky when you cook it. The red variety is high in anthocyanins, antioxidants that help stave off heart disease and diabetes. All colors are loaded with compounds that may help fight breast cancer. Cabbage is also a top source of bone-strengthening vitamin K.

How you can eat it » Eat cabbage raw: Shred it and mix with vinaigrette; the oil will help you absorb the nutrients. Or cooked: Sauté thinly sliced cabbage with chopped onions and garlic, a little olive oil and a splash of vinegar for a super side dish.

Best time to buy » Cabbage season is a long one—July through March.

Insider tip » Get an extra benefit from the friendly bacteria in cabbage's fermented form, sauerkraut. "By having a stockpile of these bugs in your digestive tract, your body's largest immune organ, you'll stay healthier," says registered dietitian David Grotto, author of *The Best Things You Can Eat.*

Nutritional tally » When it comes to calories, cabbage is about as low as you can go—just 20 calories a cup! It is also a great source of vitamins C and K.

CANTALOUPE

Why you should eat it » It puts antiaging nutrients in your fruit salad, thanks to its riches in polyphenols and beta-carotene. One study found that women who routinely ate cantaloupe had a lower risk of metabolic syndrome, a cluster of symptoms that puts you at risk for heart disease.

How you can eat it » Toss ½ cantaloupe, cubed, with ¼ c. crumbled feta cheese, 1 Tbsp. chopped fresh mint, ¼ c. chopped hazelnuts and your favorite citrus vinaigrette (makes 4 servings). Another idea: Cantaloupe *agua fresca*. Combine the juice of 2 limes and some chopped mint with a pureed, strained melon and 4 c. water and refrigerate. Serve chilled (makes 4 servings).

Best time to buy » You aren't going to find a sweet, juicy local cantaloupe in the dead of winter. The U.S. cantaloupe season runs from June through August. The rest of the year, you're depending on imports.

Insider tip » Smell the bottom of the cantaloupe, called the blossom end. If you can detect the aroma of the fruit, it's ripe. No odor means it's underripe, and an overpowering aroma says it's overripe.

Nutritional tally » One cup of melon balls is just 60 calories and gives you a significant amount of beta-carotene—30 times more than an orange—plus more than 100% of your daily requirement for vitamin C.

CITRUS FRUITS

Why you should eat them » A study involving more than 69,000 women found that those who ate several servings of citrus fruit a day had a 10% lower risk of stroke than women who ate less.

How you can eat them » All citrus foods contain fiber, which helps you feel full, making them an ideal snack for weight watchers. But pass on the juice, which can really tally up the calories and offers no fiber and no fill-you-up value.

Best time to buy » Citrus fruit is available all year, but you'll pay a premium price for it in winter if you don't shop wisely, especially for lemons and limes.

Insider tip » When you see blood oranges in the market, don't pass them up. One study found that drinking blood orange juice inhibited the accumulation of body fat.

Nutritional tally » Oranges tend to get all the glory when it comes to vitamin C, but grapefruit has more. One medium orange contains 70 milligrams of vitamin C, which nearly satisfies your daily mini-

When to Buy Organic

Yes, it costs more. "Shopping the organic aisle can cost as much as three times more than conventionally grown foods," says registered dietitian Elizabeth Somer, author of *Eat Your Way to Happiness*. So go organic for just these 12 "dirtiest" fruits and vegetables, which research shows have the highest levels of pesticide residues:

* Apples
* Bell peppers
* Blueberries
* Celery
* Cucumbers
* Grapes
* Lettuce
* Nectarines
* Peaches
* Potatoes
* Spinach
* Strawberries

Doing this alone will lower your intake of potentially dangerous pesticides by nearly 80%, according to the Environmental Working Group.

mum need, while a grapefruit has 88 milligrams. Also, don't discount the nutrition in the lemon you squirt on your fish and in your tea. The juice of one lemon meets 25% of your daily vitamin C need, and a lime offers 18%.

CARROTS

Why you should eat them » You know that bright orange color comes from beta-carotene, but here's something you may not know: Studies show that out of the vast array of veggies brimming with beta-carotene, the deepest shades of orange—namely, carrots—provide the most protection against cardiovascular disease.

How you can eat them » One study found that people significantly favored the taste of steamed carrots over boiled carrots. For more adventure, try them roasted, Italian-style: Toss carrots with olive oil and breadcrumbs, then roast with raisins and Parmesan for a sweet-savory side. Or, puree as a soup: Sauté carrots with onion, garlic and ginger; add chicken stock and simmer until tender, 10 to 15 min. Blend until smooth, stir in a splash of milk and top with diced avocado. Raw, they are the perfect snack. For a bit of a kick, shred them

She did it!

LINDSAY MICHALCIK
AGE **35**
LOST **18 POUNDS!**

HERE'S HOW: "Figuring out how to fit in exercise was key. I do a workout DVD before work a few mornings each week, and [hubby] Brendan and I have a standing gym date on Saturday and Sunday mornings. We completely changed our eating habits, too. Now we stick to one serving of protein each and load up on veggies, not unhealthy carbs. We'll still take the kids to Chuck E. Cheese, but we bring our own snacks or eat from the salad bar."

in a food processor, then toss with olive oil, lemon juice and a pinch of cumin for a simple, flavorful salad.

Best time to buy » Although they are available all year round, you'll get the most flavorful carrots when you buy them locally during the prime growing seasons of summer and fall.

Insider tip » Cooking carrots makes their beta-carotene more available to your body. Also, you'll retain the most beta-carotene by storing carrots in the refrigerator wrapped in a damp paper towel in an airtight container.

Nutritional tally » A cup of carrots offers 407% of your minimum daily need for vitamin A. The same cup comes in at only 37 calories with 3.4 grams of fiber.

CHERRIES

Why you should eat them » They are loaded with antiaging and anticancer compounds. Tart cherries (often sold as Montmorency or Balaton) are high in anthocyanin, an antioxidant with potent anti-inflammatory properties.

Frozen Trumps Fresh

Talk about a win-win! Not only do frozen vegetables save you cash and time (no chopping or prep!), they also may deliver more vitamins than fresh produce. Research has found that frozen vegetables can contain more nutrients than those found in the fresh-food aisle.

"Nutrient levels drop during shipping and as produce sits in your refrigerator," says Joanna Dolgoff, M.D., author of *Red Light, Green Light, Eat Right!* But when produce is flash-frozen at its peak, it retains more of its vitamins and flavor.

How you can eat them » Pop 'em as a snack, or pit them and sprinkle over Greek yogurt or ice cream. For dinner, halve and remove pits, then sauté with a little sugar, water and rosemary to make a cherry compote that'll snazz up any piece of meat or poultry.

Best time to buy » From late May until early August.

Insider tip » The sweetest ones are deep red with intact stems and firm, but not rock-hard, skins.

Nutritional tally » One cup (about 17 cherries) has only 87 calories, making for a great snack.

CORN

Why you should eat it » A veggie this delicious is a gift from the nutrition gods. The yellow pigment comes from carotenoids, mainly lutein and zeaxanthin, compounds that can protect your vision and prevent hardening of the arteries and possibly even cancer.

How you can eat it » We like barbecued corn on the cob: Husk and wrap each cob in foil and grill for about 10 min., turning a few times. Remove and lightly coat with equal parts low-fat mayo and fat-free plain yogurt, a pinch of chili powder and a squeeze of lime juice, then sprinkle with a little Parmesan cheese. Or, grill or steam the corn plain, then cut the kernels off the cob and toss them in salads and salsa.

Best time to buy » Nothing says summer like fresh corn on the cob! But don't be sad when the season ends. Frozen is just as nutritious as fresh. Canned corn is good, too. A Cornell University study found that cooking increases the antioxidants in corn.

Insider tip » Squeeze more corny nutrition into your diet by always buying corn tortillas. OK, so we're talking Southwestern, not Mediterranean, but who can live without a taco?

Nutritional tally » Each ear or ½ cup of kernels has about 80 calories and packs 10% of your daily fiber needs.

EGGS

Why you should eat them » They are nutritionists' number one protein source, the nutrient that's crucial to helping you feel satisfied. That makes eggs the ideal breakfast food. "Protein lowers levels of hormones that prompt hunger and boosts levels of hormones that help you feel full," says Heather Leidy, Ph.D., who led a study at the University of Missouri–Columbia that found that a protein-rich breakfast reduces cravings and overeating.

Make Room for Chocolate

You won't find chocolate on the Mediterranean food pyramid, but The Girlfriends Diet wouldn't be for us if it were dismissive of (arguably) our favorite decadent treat.

Dark chocolate got out of diet detention more than a decade ago when multiple studies found that it is brimming with healthful compounds called flavonoids that protect the heart and help prevent stroke. Now, newer research from the University of Cambridge shows that women whose diets include chocolate—dark or milk—have a 37% lower risk of heart disease than those who live in chocolate deprivation, a state of being we don't recommend.

And here's the good part: A University of Copenhagen study found that nibbling a little bit of dark chocolate helped people eat 15% less at their next meal. Milk chocolate didn't have the same effect, because it's not as satiating as the dark stuff, the researchers say.

Nevertheless, the sad reality still remains that chocolate is sinfully caloric: Just one ounce contains 155 calories and eight grams of fat, including 5¼ grams of saturated fat (the rest of the fat is mostly the good stuff).

So, the word of caution is: Take it *easy*. One of the most pleasurable ways to enjoy a piece of chocolate is as a dessert after a nice dinner out. Knowing it's waiting for you at home makes it easy to pass up the much-too-big and much-too-caloric choices on a restaurant dessert tray. Just make sure to keep it to one ounce!

One study found that morning egg eaters gobbled 330 fewer calories throughout the day than people who ate a carb-loaded meal, like a bagel. In this case, it's the seven grams of protein per egg that wards off hunger pangs later.

How you can eat them » Try them sunny-side up the way the Mediterraneans do: fried in olive oil instead of butter. Best yet for weight watchers: Hard-boil them, and eat them for a snack or slice them into a salad.

Best time to buy » The fresher, the tastier, so try this test before cracking: Place an egg in a bowl of cold water. If it rises, it's old, so ditch it! If it sinks, omelets for dinner!

Insider tip » Forget all the hoo-ha you've heard about cholesterol and eggs. That's old news. Despite the cholesterol in the yolk, a review of eight studies has found that you can eat an egg every day without raising your risk of heart attack or stroke. However, says the American Heart Association, it's a good idea to stick to two yolks a week or less if you already have high cholesterol.

Nutritional tally » For about 70 calories, one large egg delivers more than six grams of filling protein. The yolks are a good source of vitamin D and choline, a nutrient important for keeping the liver, heart and brain healthy.

WHAT THE FOOD EXPERTS SAY

"You'll find a carton of eggs in any R.D.'s fridge, including mine. There's limited evidence linking egg consumption and heart disease."
—*Jennifer McDaniel, Academy of Nutrition and Dietetics spokesperson*

FENNEL

Why you should eat it » Fennel, along with its spicy seeds, gets its licorice-like flavor from anethole, which, together with its other phytonutrients, has been found to be more potent than vitamin E at fighting off free radicals that damage cells.

How you can eat it » Slice it raw to punch up salads and sides. Add it to arugula with orange segments and a citrus vinaigrette; or toss with olive oil, salt and pepper, and bake for 30 minutes for a veggie side. Fennel seeds are a natural match for many Mediterranean diet foods, especially tomatoes, olive oil and fatty fish.

Best time to buy » Fennel likes cool weather and is at its peak in late fall and early winter.

Insider tip » You can find nutrition in all parts of the plant—the bulb, the seeds and even the fronds. You can even chop up the fronds and substitute them for basil to make pesto.

Nutritional tally » A diet delight—just 27 calories for a cup, chopped—and it has as much energy-boosting potassium as a small banana.

FISH

Why you should eat it » Fatty fish—salmon, tuna, mackerel, trout and swordfish are among the top choices—is the number one source of omega-3s, the fatty acids that can reduce your risk of heart disease and stroke, and that may even increase serotonin, a happy-mood brain chemical.

How you can eat it » Here's a simple Mediterranean-style way to make salmon that's perfect every time: Season pieces with salt and pepper and cook, skin side up, with a little olive oil in a hot pan for 1 min. Flip, cover, remove from heat and let sit for 15 min.

How to buy it » Look for wild varieties rather than farmed, and go for salmon, which generally does not have the level of mercury found in tuna. Also, select canned salmon over tuna. It's almost always wild. Or buy salmon frozen, which is also almost always wild.

Insider tip » The U.S. Environmental Protection Agency (EPA) says

Fishing for the Best Fish

An increasingly global fish market and a proliferation of choices often mean confusion for the environmentally conscious, whether you're weighing options at the fish counter or ordering from the sushi bar. David Carpenter, M.D., director of the University at Albany's Institute for Health and the Environment, reveals your safest bets among all those fish in the sea.

Shrimp: Gulf or Thai? Gulf. Southeast Asian shrimp farms have poor environmental standards.

Salmon: King or sockeye? Sockeye. King salmon live longer, accruing more contaminants. Opt for wild varieties from British Columbia and Alaska.

Canned Tuna: Albacore or light? Light. It comes from a smaller fish, so it has less mercury.

Canned Salmon: Salmon or tuna? Salmon. It's lower in mercury than tuna. Plus, it's often wild, not farmed.

the amount of mercury and other contaminants we are exposed to from eating a few servings of fish a week fall within safe levels, and both the EPA and most doctors say the benefits of eating fish far outweigh any risk. However, if you're pregnant or trying to get pregnant, play it safe and stay away from sushi and high-mercury species, like swordfish and albacore tuna.

Nutritional tally » Even fatty fish such as salmon and tuna only contain about 160 calories and about six grams of fat per four-ounce serving. Compare that with the same amount of sirloin steak at 240 calories and 112 grams of fat.

HERBS AND SPICES

Why you should eat them » They're a no-calorie way to perk up your meals and your health. "Most spices have tremendous antioxidant and anti-inflammatory effects," says Molly Kimball, R.D., nutrition director at the Ochsner Health System's Elmwood Fitness

Center in New Orleans. Also, chili peppers, ginger and turmeric have all been found to help give your metabolism a boost.

How you can eat them » With abandon! You can change the flavor of anything you cook by varying your combination of herbs and spices—very important to keeping your diet interesting.

Best way to buy » Whole spices are best, as they have a longer shelf life—about two years compared with six months. And there's no need to shell out money on expensive fresh herbs. If you don't grow your own, dried ones are fine—they actually deliver more flavor.

Insider tip » Try rosemary or turmeric in your burgers, as they are believed to be some of the most powerful antioxidants on earth. Research shows that they may counteract carcinogens, including those that may be produced during cooking. Or add oregano to your pasta sauce: Research has found that it is also full of superpotent antioxidants.

Nutritional tally » The best news yet! Herbs and spices add very few calories while taking flavor to the max. Consider them freebies.

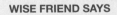

WISE FRIEND SAYS

Spice up your food to boost the burn."

Adding ginger and/or cinnamon to the food you eat raises your body temperature, so your metabolism has to speed up slightly to cool it down. A few ways to get the perk: Sprinkle a teaspoon of grated ginger into your oatmeal, smoothies and lemon-lime seltzer. Add a pinch of cinnamon to a bowl of butternut squash soup. Or add cinnamon to your coffee grounds to boost your brew.

KALE

Why you should eat it » It is today's veggie hero. A ½ cup packs 420% of your minimum daily requirement for vitamin K, a nutrient that plays a starring role in bone health. It has even more disease-fighting antioxidants than spinach.

How you can eat it » It's great in salads tossed with lemon vinaigrette. And you've got to try kale chips: Wash the leaves, remove the stems, break into bite-size pieces, pat dry with a towel and drop into a bowl. Evenly coat the kale with a teaspoon or so of olive oil and salt to taste, then arrange in a single layer on a parchment-lined baking sheet. Bake at 350°F for 10 to 15 min., until the edges are lightly browned. Crispy, salty and crazy-good for you!

Best time to buy » Grab a bunch when it's in season from November through March.

Insider tip » Although the leaves can taste a little bitter, the smaller ones are milder and more tender.

Nutritional tally » Calorie bliss! One cup of cooked kale has only 36 calories and virtually no fat, plus it has 2.6 grams of fiber. And it's packed with vitamin A, vitamin C, iron and calcium.

WHAT THE FOOD EXPERTS SAY

"If there's one veggie that every nutritionist across the country eats and recommends, it's kale. It's so nutrient-dense.
—*Carolyn Brown, R.D., Foodtrainers, New York City*

LEAFY GREENS

Why you should eat them » Their rich, deep-green color is a sign that they are flush with antioxidant carotenoids, and virtually all leafy greens are excellent sources of antioxidant vitamins A, C and E, plus the minerals iron, magnesium and potassium. Together these nutrients team up to fight heart disease, cancer, stroke and many other degenerative diseases. It's also where we can get our daily requirement for vitamin K, which protects our bones and brain, and helps guard against inflammatory disease.

How you can eat them » Like people in the Mediterranean Basin do—at practically every meal—sautéed quickly in olive oil or garlic. Some are even known to throw a fried egg onto a pile of greens for breakfast.

How you should buy them » You can save yourself the fuss of having to wash all those greens by buying them already washed and ready to eat, though they may be more expensive that way.

Insider tip » Go for micro-greens; they're like super veggies. Greens picked at seven to 14 days old have as much as 40 times more vitamins and nutrients than their more elderly (and conventionally eaten) counterparts, reports a U.S. Department of Agriculture (USDA) study. Their flavors really pop, too. But beware, they can be expensive. Generally, the darker the greens, the better they are for you. But all greens, even iceberg lettuce, are good for you.

Nutritional tally » Four cups of shredded leafy greens has only about 20 calories, so consider them a diet freebie. Just make sure to count what you add to them!

NUTS

Why you should eat them » A long-term large population study found that healthy older people who ate about an ounce of nuts a day as part of a Mediterranean diet significantly reduced their risk of stroke and heart disease—more so than people who followed the same diet sans the nuts. The reason? Their fat mostly comes from heart-healthy monounsaturates. And here's another reason to eat them: Nut lovers weigh less! Eating nuts as a snack has been shown to reduce hunger and the desire to eat between meals, with no affect on weight. In fact, nut lovers weigh on average about four pounds less than people who don't eat nuts. You shouldn't shovel them in by the handful, but studies have found that people who regularly nosh on nuts are leaner than those who don't—possibly because they're so satisfying that you end up eating less of other foods.

How you can eat them » As a daily snack. Health experts recommend an ounce of nuts a day to promote heart health.

Best kind to buy » *All* nuts are healthy, even peanuts, which are actually a legume. The healthiest way to eat them is raw and unsalted.

Insider tip » Reach for pistachios. A recent USDA study reports that our bodies don't completely absorb the fat in them. As a result, if you eat a one-ounce serving, you will take in roughly 160 calories, which is 5% less than their full caloric value.

Nutritional tally » Count out an ounce (that's about 24 almonds, 47 pistachios) and savor them slowly. An ounce of mixed nuts comes to about 175 calories with 14.5 grams of fat—nearly nine of them healthy monounsaturates and three polyunsaturates.

WHAT THE FOOD EXPERTS SAY

"Too many of my clients steer clear of nuts because they're high in fat, but dietitians eat them because we know that monounsaturates, in moderation, can help you maintain and even lose weight."

—*Keri Glassman, New York City dietitian and author of* The New You and Improved Diet

OATMEAL

Why you should eat it » Oatmeal is probably every nutritionist's favorite breakfast food, but you may not realize why: It's full of soluble fiber, a bad-cholesterol buster that also helps burn belly fat. The high amount of fiber found in oats is known to help lower total cholesterol levels.

How you can eat it » For extra nutrition without many added calories, make your oatmeal with unsweetened almond milk or soy milk, and add berries. What a wonderful way to start the day!

Best kind to buy » Go for the original steeled oats and use your own healthy add-ons. When buying other varieties, make sure to check the labels for unwanted sugar.

Insider tip » Pairing vitamin C–rich strawberries with oatmeal helps your body absorb more of the iron found in the oats.

Nutritional tally » A ½ cup of cooked oatmeal (no milk) is 120 calories and contains four grams of fiber, enough to help you stay fuller longer.

OLIVE OIL

Why you should eat it » The Mediterranean diet is considered a healthy diet, but top experts never refer to it as a *low-fat* diet. The reason is monounsaturated fat–rich olive oil. It's the food that most defines the Mediterranean diet. "Several lines of evidence point to olive oil *per se* and the olive oil–centered Mediterranean diet as conducive to better health and longevity," says Antonia Trichopoulou, M.D., Ph.D., an Athens researcher and Mediterranean diet expert. It is also the food most often associated with a reduced prevalence of chronic disease. A study published in *BMJ* also found it to be positively associated with mental health.

WHAT THE **FOOD** EXPERTS SAY

"Dietitians love it when good taste, nutrition and health meet—and extra-virgin olive oil is a triple-win.
—*Kate Geagan, M.S., R.D., author of* Go Green, Get Lean

How you can eat it » As you would butter. Get rid of the saturated fat–rich butter in your kitchen (or at least keep it in the freezer) and use olive oil in your cooking. Although olive oil has a low cooking point, the International Olive Oil Council says it's OK to sauté with it.

ᐳᐸ Cook with Better Oils ᐳᐸ

Experiment with almond oil and avocado oil, which come in second and third to olive oil in terms of their healthy monounsaturated fat content. Canola, considered another heart-healthy oil, comes in fourth. You'll still be on track using any of these healthy monos.

Best kind to buy » EVOO—extra-virgin olive oil—is your best nutritional buy. Studies show that whatever olive oil and virgin olive oil contribute to your health, extra-virgin does it even better. It's also made from the first pressing of olives, so it is purer and more flavorful.

Insider tip » Greek olive oil is believed to be superior to other Mediterranean oils, but don't buy more than you can use in a month. Studies have found that the nutritional quality of olive oil gradually starts to dissipate when it sits around longer. Also, olive oil is sensitive to high temperatures, so when sautéing, use medium heat.

Nutritional tally » Though it is super-good for you and should be your fat of choice, if you're trying to lose weight, you need to take it slowly. The 120 calories per tablespoon (20 more than butter!) can add up fast. What you get in return is 10 grams of monounsaturated fat.

PEAS

Why you should eat them » There are plenty of reasons to say, "Yes, peas!" They are loaded with a unique assortment of key antioxidants and polyphenols. Plus, they're digested slowly, which helps keep you full longer.

How you can eat them » Any way, they're delicious! Toss them into a salad, stir them into soup, or swap green peas for chickpeas in a hummus recipe and scoop with toasted pita triangles.

Best time to buy » Fresh peas are a summertime treat, but don't feel bad about getting peas from the freezer aisle. Frozen ones have as many nutrients as fresh ones.

Insider tip » Researchers suggest that peas' unusual nutritional makeup and low glycemic rating make them an important asset to regulating blood sugar and lowering the risk of type 2 diabetes. This goes for all peas: garden, snow and snap.

Nutritional tally » A ½-cup serving contains 62 calories and nine grams of fiber, plus plenty of bone-building vitamin K.

PEACHES

Why you should eat them » Because they are out-of-this-world delicious in season! Some research shows that the polyphenols found in the flesh beneath the fuzzy skin may help prevent breast cancer.

How you can eat them » Sliced over morning cereal, mixed into low-fat yogurt or atop frozen yogurt. Chop them up and add to salsa. Brush them with olive oil and grill them for a summertime dessert or as a side to grilled chicken. Slice them thin and add to iced tea. Or simply eat them whole as you might eat apples.

Greens + Fat = Nutritional Balance

Eating a big salad for lunch is one of the easiest ways to get to your recommended fill of veggies, but if you're topping it off with fat-free ranch dressing—or even just plain balsamic vinegar—you could be missing out on key vitamins, say Purdue University researchers.

They found that many cancer-fighting, heart-healthy nutrients in vegetables need to be eaten with some fat so that the body can adequately absorb them. The absolute best choice, of course, is a monounsaturated fat like olive oil. All it takes is a teaspoon (that's just 40 calories) to do the trick and allow your body to absorb the vitamins.

Best time to buy » They are grown in 47 states and are in season from May through October. If the peaches you buy are hard when you bring them home, ripen them on the counter before popping them into the fridge.

Insider tip » Buy organic if you can. Peach fuzz can help protect the fruit against bugs, but it can also collect pesticide residue, says Jackie Newgent, a Brooklyn, NY–based chef and registered dietitian.

Nutritional tally » One medium peach has just 60 calories and zero fat, with two grams of fiber, making it an ideal snack.

PLUMS

Why you should eat them » Even the ancient Romans loved plums, and here's what they didn't know: These juicy little gems are loaded with a special class of polyphenols and antioxidant vitamin A, which

So Many Milks!

Cow, soy, almond, rice, goat. (Yes, goat). There are so many ways to get your morning moo (or whatever), it begs the question: *What's best for me?*

For the dieter, the best calorie choice is almond. A full eight-ounce glass contains only 60 calories and 2.5 grams of fat. The plus side: We think it's really yummy—if you like almonds, you'll love the milk. The minus: It contains barely any protein, so make sure to get it from another source at breakfast.

The best overall choice, though, is skim cow's milk, at 83 calories, eight grams of protein and zip on the fat. One glass provides as much filling protein as a jumbo egg. Plus, it has 300 milligrams of calcium and it's a great way to get a dose of vitamin D, a nutrient most women are not getting nearly enough of.

If you're allergic to dairy or lactose-intolerant, soy and nut milks are cereal saviors. Just choose brands that are fortified with calcium and vitamin D to get some nutrients. These days, most of these types of milk are in the dairy section of your supermarket right next to "traditional" cow's milk.

your body uses to protect your eyesight, boost your immunity and keep your skin and bones healthy.

How you can eat them » They are plum-good grilled! Just quarter and then thread them onto skewers with chunks of red onion and chicken or shrimp. You could also try grilled plums over frozen vanilla yogurt for dessert. Or keep raw, pitted plums in the freezer and puree them with low-fat yogurt and one or two other fruits for a smoothie.

Best time to buy » They are in season in all their arrays of colors between May and October.

Insider tip » To pick the perfect plum, look for one that yields a bit when you poke it and feels soft at the tip. You can ripen still-hard fruits in a paper sack on your counter.

Nutritional tally » One plum has just 30 calories and one gram of fat.

POMEGRANATE SEEDS

Why you should eat them » Pomegranate seeds are considered to be a natural pharmacy of polyphenols and antioxidants that combine to reduce the risk of heart disease, cancer and stroke.

How you can eat them » As fruit goes, a pomegranate can be intimidating, even if you know to eat only the seeds. Stir them into yogurt or pancake batter (*mmm!*), serve them on top of roasted salmon or sprinkle them over pumpkin soup. Drop a few seeds into a glass of champagne, or add some juice to a martini.

Best time to buy » They're only in season from October through January, so be sure to take advantage then.

Insider tip » You can buy the seeds alone, but in season, you might want to buy the whole fruit and extract the seeds yourself, as they taste fresher. Extracting them is easy, though still a little messy, with this technique: Slice off the stem, cut the fruit into four pieces and push the seeds into a bowl of water. Skim off the pulp and strain off the water. Use packaged pomegranate juice sparingly—just a little here and there—as it tends to be high in calories and is not as nutritious as the seeds themselves.

Nutritional tally » An 80-calorie half-cup serving has as much fiber as a bowl of bran flakes.

POPCORN

Why you should eat it » It's the best food finding since chocolate was declared healthy: Three cups of popcorn contain even more good-for-you polyphenols than a serving of fruit. Because fruit contains about 90% water, it means the nutrients are also diluted. Popcorn is only 4% water, so the nutrients are concentrated. That makes it *G-O-O-D F-O-R Y-O-U*. But that doesn't mean you should ignore fruit. Just consider popcorn for a change of pace or when you're in the mood for something crunchy. It's no substitute for the nutrients you could be missing out on in fruit.

How you can eat » Make sure to skip the butter and salt to keep your kernels in the healthy zone.

Best kind to buy » Order a small, no butter, at the concession stand, or make your own air-popped or light microwave brand at home.

Insider tip » Surprise! Candied popcorn is not out of the question. You can eat a big bowl—five cups!—of Jolly Time Healthy Pop Caramel Apple popcorn at just 110 calories and two grams of fat.

Nutritional tally » A small-size bag of movie theater popcorn is around 450 calories, even without the butter, so be frugal among the unknowns. It's best to take along your own—hey, why not!—100-calorie minis. We like Orville Redenbacher's 94% fat-free microwavable SmartPop! It's only 240 calories for a whole bag—and it's big.

POTATOES

Why you should eat them » Pity the poor potato. This much-maligned food has been getting a bad rap as a diet disaster for decades, yet it is a staple of the Mediterranean diet, where potatoes are eaten almost daily. It's only been in recent years that researchers have discovered the potato's true nutritional nature: *At least* 60 different antioxidants have been identified, which puts the spud right up there with the healthiest of vegetables.

How you can eat them » What's wrong with potatoes is the way Americans like to eat them: French-fried and bathed in gobs of butter. Instead, keep it simple. Go for microwaved or steamed new potatoes (those cute little ones you see in the market). Add cubed potatoes to your soups and stews or sliced leftover red potatoes to a salad. And keep the skin intact because the nutrients are found in the flesh *and* the shell.

Best kind to buy » Potatoes marketed as "baby" or "new" potatoes are nutritionally superior to baking and white potatoes. Potatoes with purple or red flesh are especially high in antioxidants. Look for them in high-end markets.

AMAZING MAKEOVER!

Geraldine Campbell

"The better I ate, the less I craved meaty, cheesy dishes."

MY BOYFRIEND, IAN, a chef, cooks almost everything in master fat, a flavor-packed mélange of bacon grease, rendered beef fat and whatever residual drippings result from his daily culinary endeavors. It's one of the things that made me fall in love with him—well, not the master fat itself, but the fact that he cooked for me: chicken-and-dumpling soup that could cure even the worst head cold, fried pound cake à la mode. I felt loved and cared for in a way that I hadn't in years—not surprisingly, I put on 12 pounds over the course of six delicious months.

Ian prefers me with a little something extra. I, on the other hand, am less thrilled with the snugness of my skinny jeans and my math-teacher arms. But I've never been very good at dieting. In high school, I stopped eating fat entirely. In college, I went dairy-free for nearly a year. And a few years later, I had a brief go at the Atkins diet. None of these lasted very long and none had lasting results.

And it's not just me: 96% to 99% of dieters who lose weight gain it back within a year, says nutritional psychologist Marc David, founder of the Colorado-based Institute for the Psychology of Eating. Listening to experts like David is what helped turn me around. I found out that diets are largely unsuccessful because we're working against our environment: an office that encourages eating at your desk or a social life that revolves around dinner with friends. As much as I disliked being on a diet, I hated being that girl who eats only salad, feigning fullness. In other words, no fun.

It's exhausting to constantly say no, and ultimately, it's not sustainable. "When we deny, deny, deny—we swing the other way, and we binge, binge, binge." says David. Wanting to avoid the pattern of past diets, I sought out the help of a nutrition counselor whose approach—enjoying food rather than turning it into the enemy—made me feel like I might be able to lose weight and keep my boyfriend.

Sadly, saying yes doesn't mean a diet of croissants, full-fat ice cream and red wine. Not that these are forever off-limits, but experts posit that if we fill our lives with healthy foods and behaviors, we just won't want the bad stuff. For example, if I would have a nutrient-packed berry smoothie instead of skipping breakfast, I wouldn't feel tempted to raid the office kitchen for animal crackers and chips. I wasn't convinced, but I was ready to give it a try.

I cleaned my kitchen of unhealthy foods (including, yes, a jar of master fat) and filled it with leafy greens, brown rice, almond butter, a few bars of dark chocolate. I started cooking more, preparing meals like quinoa and black bean salad. It didn't taste overly healthy (by which I mean cardboard-like) and I found (truly) that the better I ate, the less I craved meaty, cheesy dishes. I felt empowered by my healthy choices, and I was bounding out of bed at 6:30 A.M., hangover-free and ready to face the day. But I wasn't sure I'd be able to stand up to the temptations when it came to making plans with friends. After a few evenings spent watching back-to-back episodes of *The Wire*, I knew being a recluse was not a long-term solution. Instead, I took one of David's suggestions and tried to mold my environment to suit me. Rather than meeting friends for indulgent meals out, I suggested going for a walk or seeing a movie. But my friends, it turns out, aren't that into long walks. My social life, then, became a series of careful calculations: If I had dinner plans, I'd eat a small lunch and run a few extra miles. If I went out for cocktails, I'd

"The calculations that initially felt exhausting became second nature."

keep it to one Negroni, a perfect sipping drink. And I gave myself nights off, too—when I'd happily indulge in carb-heavy, guilt-free meals over a bottle of Barolo. Most of the time, I felt smug and superior as I had just a bite of blueberry crumble. Other times, I felt discouraged. It turns out that saying yes to farro and healthy goodness can sometimes feel like saying no—especially when your boyfriend cooks for a living and has a pint-of-ice-cream-a-day habit and a marathoner physique.

I approached the Ian issue cautiously, explaining that while I loved his cooking, my stomach couldn't keep up with his. We talked about my fear that abstaining from his decadent feasts might make him think me a killjoy. It wouldn't, he assured me. He supported me 100%.

I've never really reached the point where I didn't want a slice of comforting pie on a cold night. I don't think I ever will. But the calculations that initially felt exhausting became almost second nature. I've also lost—and kept off—much of the courtship weight without feeling deprived. To celebrate, I let Ian make me a bison burger with cucumbers and feta—hold the master fat, please.

Insider tip » In one study, people who ate microwaved potatoes every day for four weeks as part of their regular diet didn't gain any weight, proving that potatoes don't make you fat.

Nutritional tally » One small potato contains about 120 calories and no fat (see!), and about three grams of fiber.

PUMPKIN

Why you should eat it » It's so much more than Halloween decor or Thanksgiving dessert. It's one of the richest sources of beta-carotene—the antioxidant best known to protect the heart and help fight cancer—known to woman.

How you can eat it » It's equally good and versatile sweet or savory. Stir canned pumpkin into oatmeal, yogurt and smoothies. We love

Four Ways to Get Added Nutrition

Yes, eating a lot of vegetables every day is crucial to achieving permanent weight loss and good health, but the way you prepare them can also give you an added healthful boost. Here are four tricks that will garner you a nutritional bonus, courtesy of Ruth Frechman, M.A., R.D., author of *The Food Is My Friend Diet*.

1. Add a little oil as you sauté or cook leafy greens. The good fats from the oil help your body absorb the nutrients that are released as the vegetable is heated.

2. After you mince garlic, let it sit out for 15 minutes. Research shows that exposing garlic to air once you chop it up promotes an enzyme reaction that releases cancer-fighting compounds.

3. Cut larger pieces or cook the vegetable whole. Cooking bigger sections of vegetables like sweet potatoes or summer squash exposes less of the food's surface to air and heat, which can destroy vitamins and nutrients.

4. When boiling potatoes, leave the peels on and cook them whole if possible. This will help preserve their high levels of vitamin C. Also, keep the lid on the pot so they cook more quickly (longer cooking time leads to higher loss of water-soluble nutrients like vitamin C).

pumpkin hummus: Combine one 16-oz. can chickpeas, 1 c. canned pumpkin puree, 2 Tbsp. olive oil, 2 cloves garlic, 1 Tbsp. lemon juice and 1 tsp. cumin, and blend until smooth. Use the canned puree in muffins, or chop up some pumpkin and roast it for a yummy side.

Best time to buy » Who doesn't know that pumpkins make their presence known in the fall? But it's so easy and equally nutritious out of the can, so you can have it year-round.

Insider tip » Don't throw out the seeds. They're nutritious in their own right, offering nerve-calming magnesium, blood-nourishing iron, immune-strengthening zinc and muscle-building protein. Sprinkle them sparingly on your cereal or oatmeal.

Nutritional tally » One cup is just 49 calories and has three grams of fiber with plenty of vitamins A and C. But be careful of those seeds: A quarter cup is 170 calories, so eat them judiciously.

SPINACH

Why you should eat it » It's like a multivitamin—a mighty tasty one. Spinach is packed with at least a dozen antioxidant flavonoids, which act as anti-inflammatory and anticancer agents, plus vitamins A, C and K. It's one of the highest sources of folate, the vitamin essential to preventing birth defects. And we can't forget Popeye, who likes to remind us that spinach is loaded with iron. Just one serving gives us nearly 40% of the minimum daily requirement. A classic study involving women living in New England found that those who ate the most spinach had the lowest risk of breast cancer.

How you can eat it » It's delicious as the featured green in a salad. Make a meal of it by adding a hard-cooked egg, a few steamed baby potatoes, some red onion, strawberries and a little olive oil–based dressing. Or steam it and squirt with olive oil spray.

Best time to buy » The fresh-cut spinach season is from spring through fall. When buying loose leaves, make sure to rinse well, as the leaves tend to collect dirt and sand. Bagged spinach is already washed, so there is no need to do it again.

Insider tip » Pick your bag of spinach from the front of the pile, not the back. A *Journal of Agricultural and Food Chemistry* study found that spinach exposed to light retained its nutrients, while spinach in the dark declined in nutrients—up to 30% in the case of folate.

Nutritional tally » OK, girlfriends—eat up. A cup of raw spinach is just seven calories.

SWEET POTATOES

Why you should eat them » If it's orange, its nutritional claim to fame has to be beta-carotene, but there's more to sweet potatoes than meets the color wheel. Ounce for ounce, sweets pack more vitamin A and beta-carotene than carrots. Their high-fiber content makes them diet-friendly, because you digest them more slowly than white potatoes. And studies show the nutrients in sweet potatoes dramatically suppress the chemical chain of events that causes body cells to age.

How you can eat them » They definitely don't have to be candied to be delicious. Bake them whole and serve halved, topped with Greek yogurt and cinnamon. Or make good-for-you fries: Cut a sweet potato lengthwise into ¼-in. slices, brush with olive oil, sprinkle with salt and paprika, and cook on a baking sheet at 350°F for 45 min.

Best time to buy » Sweet potatoes are at their peak—no surprise—at the end of November, just in time for Thanksgiving.

Insider tip » Those tubers you see in the store marketed as yams? They're really sweet potatoes with a firmer, mealy consistency, as opposed to the sweet softness of the ones we're most familiar with.

Nutritional tally » These orange-fleshed tubers are a nutritional bonanza: A five-ounce sweet potato has just about 100 calories and about four grams of filling fiber.

TOMATOES

Why you should eat them » The juicy news on summertime's most popular fruit (yep, it is!): A Tufts University study found that people who ate a tomato-rich diet had a significantly lower risk of heart disease than people who ate the least amount of tomatoes. And there are dozens of other studies to back it up. A study conducted at Ohio State University found that a diet rich in tomato-based foods, even for the short-term, helps protect postmenopausal women against breast cancer. The source of all this health is lycopene, the nutrient that gives the tomato its rich red color.

How you can eat them » There are oh, so many ways! Here are but a few: tucked into a grilled vegetable or turkey sandwich, a bright add-on to a summer salad and, of course, pizza, pizza, pizza. A delicious side-dish idea: Simply cut tomatoes into thick slices, top with shredded Parmesan cheese, drizzle with a little olive oil, and bake for 15 min.

Best time to buy » Summertime, when they can be plucked right from the vine. A hothouse tomato can't hold a candle to a red, juicy summer one, nutritionally or taste-wise. But don't fret in the winter. Lycopene explodes when tomatoes hit the heat, meaning canned tomato *anything* is even better.

Insider tip » The redder, the better. That deep color means they're loaded with lycopene. And never refrigerate them. Tomatoes are sunkissed and refrigeration can chill the taste right out of them. If you must refrigerate, bring to room temperature before eating or using. You'll get back some, but not all, of the flavor.

Nutritional tally » One medium-size ripe red tomato is just 20 calories with one gram of fiber.

TROPICAL FRUITS: PAPAYA, MANGO, PINEAPPLE, GUAVA

Why you should eat them » The vibrant colors of these and other fruits grown in warm climates are the giveaway that they are filled with important antioxidants and essential nutrients. Most noteworthy and common to all of them is their important dietary fiber and vitamin C content.

How you can eat them » Mix them all together for an out-of-this-world salad. Turn any or all into a salsa with diced tomato, red onion, cilantro, some spice and a shot glass of watermelon juice. Slice them alongside your morning egg, or add them to your cereal or yogurt.

Best time to buy » Exotic fruits are all imports, and your local supply depends on your area vendors.

Insider tip » Feeling a little heavy today? Eat some pineapple. It contains an enzyme called bromelain that promotes digestion and eases bloating. Papaya is another depuffer.

Nutritional tally » All this nutrition adds up to about 80 to 120 calories per cup, depending on the fruit.

Vegetable Juice: The Ultimate Diet Drink

The new diet drink of choice may be vegetable juice, report Baylor College of Medicine scientists. When they studied 81 overweight people on a diet rich in foods like fruits, vegetables, whole grains and lean meats, they found that those who drank an eight-ounce glass of low-sodium vegetable juice every day for three months lost on average three more pounds than those following the same diet but without the juice. The scientists theorized that the juice fills you up so you eat less overall.

Try sipping a glass while you are preparing dinner to help prevent premeal noshing. One cup of low-sodium vegetable juice or tomato juice contains only 50 calories and counts for two servings of vegetables, making it a great way to ratchet up your vegetable intake. Just make sure to add it into your calorie count for the day.

WATERMELON

Why you should eat it » Next to tomatoes, watermelon is the richest source of lycopene, the carotenoid that offers us protection against cancer and heart disease. An 11-year study found that people who ate the most watermelon had a 25% lower risk of coronary artery disease. And because it's 92% water, it'll help keep you hydrated on sweltering days when you're out there burning fat.

How you can eat it » Toss cubed melon with tomatoes, low-fat feta and your favorite vinaigrette. Skewer and grill it with fish and vegetables. Puree it and add it to a drink for a refreshing summer twist.

Best time to buy » Summer. When selecting a melon, compare a few that are the same size and pick the heaviest one. That means it contains more water, so it'll be juicier.

Insider tip » Always eat a bit of the white part of the rind. It contains citruline, a nutrient that improves blood flow.

Nutritional tally » Two cups of watermelon has 80 calories.

GF STAY SLIM SECRET

"Before going out to eat, I have some filling cereal. That way, unhealthy foods don't tempt me.
—*Selena A. Vincent, facebook.com/goodhousekeeping*

WHOLE GRAINS

Why you should eat them » Eating three or more servings of whole grains each day can help reduce your risk of heart disease, stroke and type 2 diabetes. But this is what you really want to hear: Studies show that people who eat them are better able to lose belly fat. One study found that women who regularly ate whole grains weighed less and had smaller waists than women who rarely ate them.

Another good reason: Research shows that your body burns more calories digesting whole grains versus the processed stuff.

How you can eat them » Bread, pasta and the multiple and much-more-interesting-than-brown-rice grains such as farro and quinoa all count (just to name a few). Go for tabouleh, a Mediterranean bulgur-wheat salad made with tomatoes and cucumber. Whip up an instant version and just add a little feta. Yum!

Best way to buy » If it's whole grain (wheat, oats, rye, etc.), the grain in the ingredients list will be preceded by the word *whole* or *whole-grain* as the first ingredient. *And* put it back on the shelf if you see the words "enriched wheat," which is code for refined white flour, or if you see a lot of words you can't pronounce. Chemical-sounding words can be translated as "processed."

Insider tip » Transition to whole grains by following the "half" rule: In pasta dishes, start out by using half whole-grain and half white. Mix your regular cereal with ½ cup of a high-fiber variety, at least three grams of fiber per serving.

Nutritional tally » Grains are good for you, and even though they contain little fat, they can be caloric, so check the label. A half cup typically contains at least 100 calories or more. But they are full of fiber, so make sure to eat something grainy at every meal.

WHAT THE FOOD EXPERTS SAY

"Most nutritionists reach for quinoa over brown rice or wheat pasta because it's a complete source of protein, which means it has all the essential amino acids your body needs."
— *Jennifer McDaniel, Academy of Nutrition and Dietetics spokesperson*

WINE

Why you might want to drink it » People who drink in moderation outlive teetotalers and alcohol abusers. Wine contains more than 500 active substances, but one in particular has been the focus of scientific scrutiny: a polyphenol called resveratrol. Some scientists believe that resveratrol works in synergy with other antioxidants to alter blood chemistry in ways that help lower cholesterol and prevent other processes that lead to cardiovascular disease. However, a recent John Hopkins University study on resveratols found no association with longevity or decreasing cardiovascular disease. While drinking is generally believed to increase the risk of breast cancer, researchers at Cedars-Sinai Medical Center found that drinking *red* wine, but not white, in moderation may reduce at least one of the risk factors for the disease.

How you can drink it » All the health benefits of drinking are attained only by drinking in moderation—for women that's a five-ounce glass a day. And no, seven in one night once a week doesn't work. The more you drink, the more risk you accumulate in other areas of health.

Best kind to buy » Red trumps white, though both offer health benefits. Heart-protecting polyphenols are concentrated in the skin of the grape and in the seeds, which are used in making red wine, but are removed when making white wine.

Insider tip » Teetotaler? That's OK. Grapes may not offer as much resveratrol as wine does, but they are considered a great nutritional snack.

Nutritional tally » A five-ounce glass of red wine contains 120 calories—another reason to keep a cap on it.

WINTER SQUASH

Why you should eat it » Squash is such an unfortunate name for a veggie that does beautiful things for your body. Yes, these orange-centric vegetables—acorn, butternut, hubbard, etc.—are packed with beta-carotene, but let's not forget that they also contain immune-boosting vitamins A and C to fend off colds.

GF WANTS TO KNOW

What's the one unhealthiest food I should never eat?

—Melissa Nudell, 49, Fargo, ND

Dear GF,

Anything white that's not a fruit, vegetable, egg, dairy or fish is a definite diet no-no. It's a sign that the food has been processed down to a very simple carbohydrate that probably doesn't have many nutrients. All GFs should help their other GFs wean themselves off this one!

How you can eat it » As a main-course entrée! Slice an acorn or butternut squash in half lengthwise, spoon out the seeds, stuff each half with brown rice, bulgur or a grain mixed with cranberries, and bake at 350°F for 30 minutes. Got leftovers? Puree with some chicken broth for a creamy low-cal soup.

Best time to buy » In winter.

Insider tip » Even though vitamin C tends to leach out when the flesh is exposed to air, it's still OK to buy it precut, as you're not losing that much nutritionally given how much you gain in additional convenience.

Nutritional tally » One cup of winter squash is about 100 calories and contains a filling nine grams of fiber.

YOGURT

Why you should eat it » Yogurt is the food most strongly linked to long-term weight loss. In a study that followed 120,000 adults for four years, people who ate at least a serving a day dropped almost a pound every four years. Those who didn't eat yogurt *gained* weight.

Research also shows that probiotics, the "good" bacteria found in yogurt, may be the reason. "Scientists have found that obese people have more of a certain type of bacteria that is more efficient at extracting energy from food," says Gerard Mullin, M.D., a gastroenterologist at Johns Hopkins Hospital. "It's possible that the 'good' bacteria in yogurt help counter these 'bad' weight-gain-causing bacteria."

How you can eat it » Just so, or mixed with fruit and churned into a smoothie.

Best kind to buy » Greek yogurt, classic yogurt with the whey strained out, is thicker and creamier. However, any yogurt will do as long as it's rich in probiotics. Look for "live and active cultures" on the container's label.

Insider tip » Greek yogurt is even *more* filling and slimming, thanks to the fact that it contains more protein (15 grams per six-ounce serving) than the classic variety. That's more than a chicken cutlet! However, dieters beware: Always go for the nonfat variety, as full-fat Greek can contain up to 70 more calories per cup.

Nutritional tally » A serving of nonfat Greek yogurt is about 100 calories. The straining that makes it thicker more than doubles the protein, from eight or nine grams to 18 or 20 grams, though calcium drops from 30% to 20%.

GF Action Plan

DO A PANTRY SURVEY. Do you have essential Girlfriends Diet Food Basket staples like beans, whole wheat pastas, grains, canned tomatoes and olive oil? Add these pantry essentials to your shopping list (see box on page 94).

PICK A FEW NEW FOODS TO TRY. Get familiar with the list in this chapter and pick out one new healthy food to try every week.

Thicker Shake, Thinner You

A liquid breakfast, really? Yep! A British study found that when people perceived a blended drink as feeling thicker, they were more likely to feel full and satisfied. And since the prospect of a full belly can quell appetite and influence portion sizes, you just might end up eating less. Good thickeners for your smoothies, but not your belly: nonfat Greek yogurt and frozen fruit.

Expanding the selection of foods you serve at home will keep your diet more interesting. Share your experiences—and recipes—with your diet club girlfriends.

REMEMBER YOUR COLORS AT EVERY MEAL. A great way to quickly see that you have enough fruits and vegetables in your meal is to make sure that every plate includes as many vibrant colors as possible—especially green, red and yellow.

✽ Order a copy of *The Girlfriends Diet* for your friend at goodhousekeeping.com/girlfriends.

✽ Share your success stories and get more dieting tips on our Facebook page at facebook.com/girlfriendsdiet.

chapter 5
Strategies That Feed Success

LOSING WEIGHT WOULD BE A BREEZE if dieting didn't make us so hungry. Or does it—*really*?

You know that on The Girlfriends Diet there is *plenty* to eat—lots of good fill-her-up breads, beans, fruits, vegetables and other super-nutritious and tasty food like avocados, almonds and salmon. The real challenge is: How am I going to squeeze it all in throughout the day? You also know there is no food that's off-limits forever. *Yes,* there are limitations, but you now understand that eating too much of the wrong foods and not enough of the right foods is, for the most part, what made your weight go up, up, up in the first place.

So why, then, do you still want to take a handful of M&M's when the bowl is passed around the conference room? Or even look at the dessert menu when you're already full from the lunch you just had with your gal pals? Or ask the bartender for just one more when you know the glass of wine you just had should be your limit? Or finish what's left on your kid's plate after you've already cleaned your own? Or mindlessly lift another pig-in-the-blanket from the hors d'oeuvres tray as it passes by at a party after you've already had three?

The reason we reach for food when we're really not hungry, say experts in behavioral weight loss, is habit. "Habits are 45% of our daily life," says David Neal, Ph.D., a psychologist and founding partner at Empirica Research, a communications and technology research firm. "They cause us to disregard rational or motivational drivers and instead be cued by context, automated actions, time pressure and low self-control."

Studies confirm that a lot of the eating we do is driven by habit rather than hunger. Researchers at the University of Southern California demonstrated this with a group of people who unknowingly were given bags of stale popcorn in two different environments: a movie theater and a conference room. While sitting watching the movie they gobbled it up—after all, what's a movie without popcorn? But in the boardroom, the stale flavor turned the group off, and they passed on it—nobody munches on popcorn at a serious business meeting anyway.

The reason diets fail or people eventually regain the weight they lose is because people haven't changed their mind-set around food, says Judith S. Beck, Ph.D., author of *The Beck Diet Solution*. It's our long-ingrained mental programming that makes us reach for a cookie just "because it's there" or continue to finish a large plate of food when half would have been just fine. The key to sticking to a weight-loss plan and making the success permanent is all a matter of mind-set. "You need to train your brain to change your mental habits," Beck says. And what that takes is practice.

SMASH THAT DIET MENTALITY. Remember, The Girlfriends Diet is a lifestyle change, something that will change your weight permanently in a natural way; it is not a diet you go on and off, then back on again. "In the past when I was 'on a diet,' one little setback meant I was suddenly 'off my diet,'" says Lisa Lillien, founder of the Hungry Girl brand and hungrygirl.com, who dropped 25 pounds and kept it off by changing her relationship with food. "Then I'd throw in the towel and tell myself I'd start again next Monday." Not ideal!

Rather, Beck suggests in her book, come up with a purpose for your desire to lose weight that will talk back to you—something you can write down and put in a prominent place, like your Girlfriends Diet Club pledge (see page 21)—that will help train your brain into a new way of thinking. Your new mantra could go something like this: *The Girlfriends Diet is not a "diet" in the traditional sense. It is a healthy lifestyle adjustment and the way I'm going to eat for the rest of my life.* Or it might be more personal: *I am choosing to make the changes required by The Girlfriends Diet because I want to be able to be healthy enough to run after my kids and join my husband when he plays tennis.* Repeat it to yourself daily and whenever needed, like when you walk up to the deli counter to order a turkey sandwich and that little voice in your head starts screaming, *But the*

She did it!

KARA GIANNECCHINI,
AGE **30**
LOST **21 POUNDS!**

HERE'S HOW: "I didn't even realize I'd ditched all my healthy habits after getting married until I woke up one day and none of my dress pants fit. Not to mention I was offered a seat on the subway—and I wasn't pregnant! I tended to turn to food for comfort, so I needed to find new ways to de-stress.

"I cut way down on sugar. Honestly, the less I have sweets, the less I want them. I'd always used food for comfort, but I don't do that anymore. I was so worried about what people might think of me after I gained the weight that I avoided making plans. I've stopped hiding out, and my husband and I have more fun together now."

corned beef special sounds so good! Go ahead, before you read any further, and write down your own mantra. Now find a special place to put it so that you will see it every day as a cue to yourself to repeat and it use daily.

"When I'm tempted to eat out of boredom, I tell myself to wait until after I complete a task. Then I get busy and usually forget about it!"
— *Trish Dunlap, Chico, CA*

PICK THE RIGHT ROLE MODEL. You can also choose an inspirational photo to boost your diet resolve. Skip shots of too-thin models and pick those of more achievable figures. Two studies found that unrealistic images can derail your efforts and may even cause weight gain. Put the photo someplace that you look at frequently and consider moving it from time to time so you won't start overlooking it.

RECOGNIZE THAT YOU CAN'T BE PERFECT ALL OF THE TIME. Celebrations and indulgences are part of life—a happy one. "If you make good choices 80% of the time, you can loosen the reins a bit the rest of the time," coaches Lillien. "You won't feel restricted, but you won't go overboard, either. So much better than black-and-white thinking."

TAKE IT ONE HABIT AT A TIME. You accumulated your bad habits around food over a lifetime, so you can't expect to overcome them overnight. As you continue reading, several of these saboteurs will resonate with you. Pick one or two of the toughest ones and start working on them. Once you feel you've formed a new healthy habit to replace an old bad habit, move on to others. Taking on too much at one time will only start to feel stressful. And you know where that leads—right to the freezer door.

TAKE IT ONE DAY AT A TIME. Stop daydreaming about the skinny jeans you'd like to slip into. Instead, keep your sights on the day-to-day steps in the process of weight loss—like making a delicious Greek salad. In a group of 126 overweight women trying to shed pounds, those who concentrated most on daily to-dos were more likely to succeed than those whose attention was on their slimmer future selves. "Focusing on the 'how' gives you concrete behavior guidance," explains study coauthor Alexandra M. Freund, Ph.D., of the University of Zurich. And the good habits you practice will help keep the pounds off.

EAT SLOW AND SAVOR. Most experts agree that the most important thing everyone needs to learn when establishing good eating habits is to eat more slowly. That means eating *mindfully*, says Beck. Think about the task at hand—eating—and actually *experience* the taste. By appreciating the food and eating more slowly, you'll actually eat less than if you just start shoveling it in and wolfing it down. Put your fork or spoon down after every bite and chew 20 times. Research shows that s-l-o-o-w eating can slash calorie intake by 10%.

"I eat the same breakfast and lunch every day, so I don't have to make food choices when I'm hungry."
— *Jane Trambley, Sharon, PA*

UNDERSTAND WHAT'S INVOLVED IN MAINTAINING YOUR WEIGHT LOSS. In a get-skinny twist, Stanford University researchers wondered if learning maintenance strategies, like the ones you are reading about in this chapter, *before* dropping pounds would help people keep off lost weight. They put one group of women on a traditional five-month-long plan followed by eight weeks of keep-it-off problem-solving sessions. Another group practiced behavioral-maintenance techniques, like daily weigh-ins and behavior-modification strategies, before they began. Everyone lost about 17 pounds, but the maintenance-first group proved to be less likely to regain what they'd lost, adding back just three pounds, while the standard dieters went up about seven. So keep reading!

KEEP TRACK OF WHAT YOU EAT. We said this earlier, but it bears repeating: Keeping a food diary or journal is the number one strategy for successful weight loss. One study, for example, tracked nearly 1,700 dieters who conscientiously wrote down everything they ate and drank and calibrated the calories. They ended up losing twice as much weight as dieters who followed the same diet but didn't keep a journal.

JOURNAL YOUR FEELINGS. Keeping a food diary can be an eye-opener as to what and how much you eat, but it can also be very revealing about your thought processes. Don't just write down what you eat; also write *about* how you're feeling about the food choices you make and the hunger cues you experience throughout the day, says Beck. You have to know your mental saboteurs if you want to outsmart them. Here's also a good place to record your mantra, as well as your daily to-dos, that will help keep your new eating lifestyle on track.

GF STAY SLIM SECRET

"I keep dark-chocolate Dove Promises in the fridge. They get hard when they're cold, so they take longer to nibble."

—*Jean Henry, Parsippany, NJ*

TALK YOURSELF OUT OF TEMPTATION. Trying to resist temptation? Here's a cool trick some girlfriends swear by: When you see the fried mozzarella balls passing by on the party platter, touch your fingers to your thumb, one at a time, while saying to yourself: *This. I. Do. For. Me.*

SAY "OK—BUT LATER." Have a fierce urge for a chocolate doughnut? Tell yourself you'll eat it—later. Any mother will recognize the power of distraction and postponement, and it turns out that research backs it up, too. Researchers from the University of Houston Bauer College of Business found that people who crave a snack, like chips or chocolate, end up wanting it less and can avoid eating it if they postpone indulging to a vague time in the future. "This helps you forget about the food in the first place because your craving usually goes away," says study coauthor Vanessa M. Patrick, Ph.D.

GF STAY SLIM SECRET

"I brush my teeth soon after I get home, and it makes me not want to eat while I prep dinner. I'll do that at night, too, so I won't eat late."
—*Angela Detwiler Zamora,*
facebook.com/goodhousekeeping

THINK BEFORE YOU EAT. When you're at a party and the hors d'oeuvres platter crosses your path, or when you're out to dinner and getting dangerously close to ordering the wrong thing, pause and ask yourself: *Do I really want to eat this? Is it really worth the calories?* It's the best way to stop yourself from mindlessly munching, says Lillien.

Outsmart the Saboteurs

Eating healthy and smart food shopping are like everything else that leads to success. You've got to plan and be prepared for the curveball that likely will come heading your way.

KEEP A SNACK STASH AT THE READY. You don't want to learn this the hard way and end up devouring a family-size bag of potato chips on your way home from the supermarket because you went food shopping on an empty stomach. If you have an emergency snack stash at the ready, you won't find yourself super-hungry between meals, and you won't fall prey to the voice in your head that says, *McDonald's is just around the corner*. Keep items such as nuts, dried fruit, plain cereal, trail mix and whole-grain crackers, proportioned in 100-calorie baggies, in your handbag, briefcase, car or gym bag.

THINK OF CALORIES IN TERMS OF RUNNING THEM OFF. Would that Philly cheesesteak seem less appealing if you knew that you'd have to hoof it for a good seven miles just to walk it off? Knowing what a dish costs in terms of burning calories rather than just knowing the calorie count has much more of an influence over whether you order

AMAZING MAKEOVER!
Linda Richards
"Healthy food choices and exercise cut my weight in half."

BY THE TIME I was 24, I had three kids and my weight had skyrocketed to over 250 pounds. After a battle with thyroid cancer (I was declared disease-free in 2001) and a devastating job loss in 2010, my weight was close to 320. My self-esteem was the lowest it had ever been, and my weight was at its highest.

I decided I could no longer "diet" because that implied I would eventually go back to my old ways.

Instead, I needed to change my *life*. I decided that if I was going to make a lifestyle change, no food could be off-limits—I simply tried to make more healthy choices, like eating fewer refined carbs and more vegetables. I also knew I needed to exercise. I wasn't comfortable going to a gym at first, so I used at-home DVDs. Once I shed 20 pounds, I felt ready to join a fitness center. I was nervous about using equipment in

front of others, so I went late at night when it was less crowded. I didn't want my discomfort stopping me from exercising. That's where I found the sign for a Biggest Loser contest and signed up for the start in January 2011. The competition was a great motivator! We were all in it together, just like on TV. We all wanted to win, but we all wanted everybody to be a winner and lose the weight they wanted to. After 16 weeks, I had lost a salad or the cheesesteak, according to one study.

When diners were given menus that included the minutes of brisk walking needed to burn off each item, they ate about 100 fewer calories than when menus offered no extra information. Listing calorie count alone—also tested in the study—didn't help people restrain themselves, so it's better to think about your favorite treats in terms of exercise costs.

Want help with the math? The calorie converter app by athlete inme.com calculates the amount of biking, swimming, jogging or walking you need to do to work off up to 4,000 items.

over 20% of my body weight—and I won first place!

By now I was *really* motivated, but still had a ways to go. My husband suggested we get into biking, since jogging was too hard on my knees. I was hooked—it felt like time flew by when I was pedaling. In June 2012, we signed up for a 100-mile bike ride to raise money for the American Diabetes Association. As I trained for the event—and tracked my activities and what I ate—the pounds kept

"I give most of the credit for my success to my support group—my family."

coming off.

I give most of the credit for my success to my support group—my family. My husband was by my side the entire way. He made healthy choices, too, and lost 65 pounds. My children (now ages 21, 18 and 16) also encouraged me to keep going with my new lifestyle.

Having those daily cheerleaders (and accountability reminders) was crucial for me. My new weight is really just the cherry on top of how much better I feel. I tell everyone: If I can do it, you can, too. Just stop making excuses—and start getting healthy!

"If you have faith, lean on whatever higher power you believe in. Pray for strength. Of course, planning ahead helps, too, especially if you're eating out."

—*Rev. Felicia Bagneris,* Good Housekeeping reader, Los Angeles, CA

CUT YOUR GROCERY CART IN HALF. *Plop, plop*—there goes the bag of cookies into the shopping basket. *Fizz, fizz*—there goes the soda pop. How many times have you sworn to buy only healthy foods at the supermarket only to come home with bags of Oreos and Cheez Doodles? Next time, try this surprisingly simple and proven-to-work tactic:

Imagine a line drawn down the center of your cart, and designate one whole side for fruit and vegetables, and the other side for everything else. In one study, women who tried this—they had a piece of tape laid through their carts to cordon it off—bought *102% more produce*! That's the way to go, girlfriends! What's more, they didn't spend any more money than usual and ended up bringing home less junk food overall.

"The tape may have acted as a constant reminder, so buying fruits and veggies was always top of mind," says Collin Payne, Ph.D., a coauthor of the study and assistant professor of marketing at New Mexico State University in Las Cruces. Breaking out the duct tape may get you some strange stares at the grocery store—thankfully, drawing a mental divider works, too.

LIMIT FOOD FRENEMIES. Just because a food is healthy doesn't mean it's your ticket to overindulge. Remember, you can have anything as long as you eat it responsibly, and that includes good-for-you but high-calorie Mediterranean-style foods like olive oil, avocado, nuts and even whole-grain breads. Calories are still critical, even when they spell *h-e-a-l-t-h-y*. "They are not a get-out-of-jail-free card!" says Jim Karas, author of *The Petite Advantage Diet.* You always need to think of your input in terms of your output—your daily calorie limit, he cautions.

REDEFINE YOUR IDEA OF FAST FOOD. Healthy food can be fast food, too. Pick up a rotisserie chicken, a bag of salad and 90-second microwavable brown rice, and you'll have a well-balanced meal that's ready in less than five minutes, says Madelyn Fernstrom, Ph.D., author of *The Real You Diet*. You'll wait longer than that in line at Arby's!

GF WANTS TO KNOW

There are so many cereals on the supermarket shelves that sound healthy until you pick them up and read the calories. For one, the high-fiber cereals always look like they are too high in calories. It just gets so confusing! How can I tell if a cereal is meeting the needs of a perpetual dieter like me? Any recommendations?

—Morning Muncher, 51, in Wyomissing, PA

Dear GF,

For starters, go for cereals that have no more than six grams of sugar and at least three grams of fiber. Also important: Make sure the *first* ingredient listed is whole-grain *something*—wheat, oats, whatever.

All the major cereal companies have made a commitment to reduce sugar and increase whole grains in their products, so finding something within these guidelines that you'll love shouldn't be too hard. To help you out, here are some GF favorites you can try:

* **Multi-Grain Cheerios.** The lightly sweetened blend of five whole grains, including oats and whole-grain corn, is tasty enough to eat out of the box. **Calories:** 110 per cup
* **Kashi Honey Sunshine.** It's hard to believe these deliciously sweet pillows pack 20 grams of whole grain and five grams of fiber. **Calories:** 100 per ¾ cup
* **Wheat Chex.** Talk about crunchy—this oldie but goodie stands up to milk. And with six grams of fiber and five grams of protein, it's a filling choice. **Calories:** 160 per ¾ cup

TURN OFF THE TUBE. TV time turns up big-time in winter when days grow short and nights are cold. Dozens of studies have linked couch potato time with unwanted pounds. Aim to keep screen time under two hours a day. In one study, people who slashed their TV-watching by roughly 50% to an average of 1.9 hours a day burned 120 more calories daily, mostly as a result of puttering around the house.

PASS ON THE "DIET" FOOD. A better strategy: Eat the right amount of the real thing instead. Packaged, faux-fat, artificially sweetened, no-cal grub may not help you shed pounds, say researchers from Beth Israel Deaconess Medical Center and Harvard Medical School, who found that people who used diet products were less likely to achieve their weight-loss goals. One reason, researchers suspect, is that when we're eating a food we consider virtuous, we're likely to eat more of it. They call this the "health halo" effect.

GET AN EYE FOR SIZE. Talk about sabotage. Housewares manufacturers are not doing us any favors by pushing oversize plates and

Tweet More, Weigh Less

If you want to be trim, get social. In a weight-loss study at the University of North Carolina at Chapel Hill, researchers discovered that the more men and women post on Twitter, the more pounds they lose. The microblogging site allows for accountability, provides support and helps people stay focused on their goals, says study author Brie Turner-McGrievy, Ph.D.

To get started, you and the girlfriends in your diet club should all get Twitter accounts and get active—follow each other, but also follow weight-loss bloggers, nutritionists and exercise gurus. The professionals will offer strategies that may help you, while your pals will help inspire you to make the right choices, celebrate victories and help you get back on track if you've had an off day. And along the way, you'll meet other dieters, making your circle of girlfriends that much bigger and stronger—with more opportunities to give and get support and to celebrate milestones.

bowls, according to research by Brian Wansink, Ph.D., at Cornell University, because it skews our perception of serving size. During the past 20 years, the average size of a dinner plate has grown from 10 inches to 12 inches or more—and our calorie intake has gone up 22%. Consider the salad plate the new dinner plate. Or just be old-fashioned and pick up an old set of dishes with eight-inch dinner plates at a flea market.

"I like to keep a pitcher of water and a small bowl of fruit on my desk. When I feel the need to snack, I have a drink first. If that doesn't do it, I reach for the fruit."

—*Karen Doyle, 45,* Good Housekeeping *reader, Amherst, NH*

STOCK UP ON FROZEN LOW-CAL ENTRÉES. Home alone with no reason to cook? Don't get caught hungry with your finger on speed dial to the local pizza parlor. Always keep a stash of healthy low-cal frozen entrées in the freezer. That way you'll always have a delicious calorie-controlled meal at the ready on those days when time gets tight and you just aren't prepared to cook.

FIND THE SWAPS YOU LOVE. Become an expert at always being on the lookout for better-for-you alternatives to decadent foods. Invite your girlfriends over for a fun afternoon of taste-testing. Have everyone bring a new lightened-up product find, and you can all see what's worth it and what's not.

READ NUTRITION LABELS. Before tossing a packaged food into your grocery cart, check its label. Women shoppers who read nutrition-facts panels weigh an average of 8.6 pounds less than those who simply grab and go.

PUT DIVERSITY IN YOUR CUPBOARD. When you write down your shopping list, add a couple of new foods from The Girlfriends Diet

Food Basket list. "Diversity is essential to a healthy diet," says Janet Brill, R.D., Ph.D., the author of *Cholesterol Down*. "The more variety you have, the greater number of nutrients your body gets." Some healthy swaps to try: Replace rice with protein-packed quinoa, peanut butter with cashew butter, and mayo with guacamole or fiber-rich hummus.

DRESS FOR SUCCESS. Say good-bye to the days of *Oops, I drowned my salad in Italian dressing*. Spray dressings are, hands down, the best way to get a controlled amount of dressing onto your greens. It's as easy as pressing a button. Ten shots at only one calorie a spritz should do the trick.

CUT UP YOUR FOOD. It's so worth the 30 seconds it takes to slice before you bite into an apple or even a piece of fried chicken. "Cutting up your food before you dig in can help you eat less," says Devina Wadhera, Ph.D., of Arizona State University. When you see more pieces of food, your mind can be fooled into thinking you've had a bigger portion, her research shows. We like them apples!

DITCH THE CANDLELIGHT. Sure, mood lighting seems romantic—until your favorite LBD no longer fits. One study from the University of Illinois found that keeping the lights dim lowered people's eating inhibitions, so they ate more than if the lights had been brighter. They were also more likely to linger at the table and continue noshing. Music choices factor in, too: Anything with a really slow tempo may also lead to loitering at the table—and eating beyond the point of being full, says Koert van Ittersum, an associate professor of marketing at the Georgia Institute of Technology in Atlanta. Meanwhile, fast tunes could speed up eating, causing you to down more.

Slicing Calories at the Pizza Palace

The kids are clamoring for you to take them out for pizza—so-o-o-o you say to yourself, *Pizza's Mediterranean, right?* Well, yes, but...a Mediterranean pizza is a lot different from the pizza we're used to. There are no Chicagoland thick crusts or gobs of double cheese oozing off the plate. Rather, Mediterraneans have a way of loving pizza that shaves *lots* of calories off the Americanized pie and that is much more nutritious. Here's how to do the same stateside:

Think thin. Make it a rule to go for thin-crust pizza only. It's crispy and yummy and will save you a good 150 calories per slice over deep-dish pizza.

Go vegetarian. Get more flavor and a lot of nutrition by adding on Mediterranean-style veggies—onions, bell peppers, black olives, spinach, whatever—instead of sausage, pepperoni and other meats. The more veggies you have, the less room there is for cheese. Just steer clear of eggplant, as it is likely it will be fried or drenched in oil. If you absolutely must have something meaty, ask for chicken.

Go easy on the cheese. Ask the pizza guy to give you *half* the cheese. Every quarter cup you cut back will save you 85 calories.

Spice it up. It'll slow you down—which might make you eat less. Strong flavors tend to make you eat more slowly and help keep you satisfied longer. Add zero-calorie zest by sprinkling on some garlic and/or onion powder, oregano and crushed red pepper.

Say no to pesto on pizza. Pesto sauce is super-healthy, but not a good idea when you're craving pizza on a diet. Pesto comes in at 275 calories for just a quarter cup, while the same amount of red sauce is only around 20 calories. So use it as an accent but not in place of the red sauce.

"If I eat a big meal, I make sure the next one is small."

—*Lisa Wilson Grant,* Good Housekeeping *reader, Norwalk, CT*

SEE RED, EAT LESS. People ate 40% less when served food on a red plate versus a blue or white one, according to research published in the journal *Appetite*. "Red usually signals 'danger' or 'stop,' and we believe these associations are what caused people in the study to not eat as much," says study coauthor Oliver Genschow from the department of social and economic psychology at the University of Basel in Switzerland.

GET A GOOD NIGHT'S SLEEP. You'll be glad you did, say researchers from the Mayo Clinic who studied the effect of sleep on eating patterns. When participants got only two-thirds of their usual amount of sleep, they ate an average of 549 more calories each day. One possible explanation is that sleep deprivation can trigger a surge of the hormones that set your appetite in motion. Tired people not only are more likely to nosh, but also take larger servings of their not-so-healthy nibbles. And remember what you learned in Chapter 2: Lack of sleep also negatively affects your metabolism. So hit the hay early, and consider it your dream diet.

Kid-Proof Your Diet

Being a mom comes with health benefits—lots of feel-good oxytocin from the cuddles, the reduced risk of breast cancer (yes, really)—but a new study from the University of Minnesota Medical School points out that there are some sneaky diet traps mothers can fall into. Stay out of them:

DIET TRAP NO. 1: You clean your kid's plate. "Calories add up quickly. The moms in our study easily took in 300 more calories per day than women without kids," says study author Jerica Berge, Ph.D. That could just be two leftover nuggets, but in a year's time, it can add up to 31 pounds. Forget the baby fat—it's the kid fat that really gets you!

Tell yourself: *I am* not *a human garbage disposal*. Don't feel bad about tossing your kid's uneaten leftovers if they can't be saved for another day.

DIET TRAP NO. 2: You replace sleep with sugar. In her study, Berge found that moms drink more sugary beverages than women who don't have kids. Why? It may be because sweetened drinks are around the house, and when you're exhausted, you use them to fuel up. If you need a jolt, switch to antioxidant-rich green tea instead. Or keep a ready supply of bottled water close by. Even mild dehydration can sap energy, so make sure to drink plenty of water.

DIET TRAP NO. 3: Stress is your co-parent. Your many roles—nurse, chauffeur, mediator—can leave you frazzled and lower your resilience to eat properly. Chronic stress also lowers your defenses against germs and viruses, and may increase your risk of depression. It may

TIPS FROM THE PROS

"I carry inspiring quotes and pictures for when I'm tempted to cheat and need a boost."
—*Sue Brown, member of the National Weight Control Registry*

"I survey the buffet for lean proteins like shrimp cocktail."
—*Kim Larson, R.D., Seattle-based dietitian*

"I eat a little bit of the seasonal treats I love and savor every bite."
—*Susan Albers, Psy.D., author of* Eat Q.

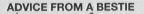

even release chemicals that help you store fat. "We need to fit in self-care, even if it's just taking a shower with the door locked or getting a manicure," Berge says. You could also squeeze in some exercise each day. Even 20 minutes of yoga or walking can be a near-instant anxiety-buster."

"In restaurants, I taste what my family orders and then stick to my healthy choice."
—*Connie Grismer,* Good Housekeeping *reader, Chandler, AZ*

How to Avoid Holiday Weight Gain

Turkey, stockings, that jolly guy in the red suit—these things are supposed to be stuffed during the holidays. You? Not so much. Yet from late October through December, you're faced with heaps of Halloween candy, the Thanksgiving splurge, holiday cakes and cookies... and party, party, party. It may seem impossible to make it to the New Year without gobbling up every last delectable goodie. Well, give yourself the best holiday gift—a plan to enjoy your favorite holiday treats through the season so you don't come out the other side of January 1 with extra padding.

Watch out for ▸ Prefestivity Feasting

It's your turn to do the entertaining and you think a taste here, a sample there while doing the cooking doesn't sound so dangerous. But if you're not careful, you could easily consume a few hundred calories before the first guest walks through the door. To keep a lid on preparty picking:

EAT BEFORE YOU COOK. Don't even think about setting foot in the kitchen to whip up your famous pecan pie on an empty stomach, warns Leslie Bonci, M.P.H., R.D., author of *The Active Calorie Diet.* It's like going food shopping when you're hungry.

Have a balanced meal or snack—one that includes girl-friendly vegetables, lean protein, healthy fats and whole grains—before

WISE FRIEND SAYS

Make mealtime family time at least once a day."

Yes, research does show that kids who gather around the table with their families for evening meals are more likely to have a healthier diet and are less likely to experiment with alcohol and drugs. But this girl-friendly piece of advice is for all you crazy-busy moms: There's nothing magical about dinner on its own. Experts say that what matters most are quality conversations and interactions between parent and child at any hour of the day. So, just make the most of breakfast, the car ride to school or story time at night.

cooking, so you won't be as tempted to nibble. A bowl of oatmeal or other whole-grain cereal with low-fat or almond milk, fruit and nuts, or a salad tossed in olive oil and vinegar and topped with grilled chicken are a few good options.

"At a buffet, I take a tablespoon of each food I want—to get a taste without too many calories."
—*Beth Evanko,* Good Housekeeping *reader,*
Warriors Mark, PA

TALLY YOUR TASTES. "If you have to sample something, put it on a plate first," Bonci says. Eating right out of the pot or pan makes it easy to lose track of how much you're consuming. A great way to keep tabs: Use a new spoon for each sample, then count the spoons as you go. Visual reminders are powerful. Research found that people ate more at an all-you-can-eat restaurant when their plates were cleared from the table between helpings than when the remnants were left in front of them.

KEEP HEALTHY SNACKS ON HAND. "Cherry tomatoes and seedless grapes—they're easy to prepare, low in calories, and they'll keep your mouth busy while you cook," Bonci says.

Watch out for ▶ Lingering Leftovers

To avoid eating like it's still a party once the guests are long gone, you should:

HAND OUT DOGGIE BAGS. "If you have extra food or caloric dishes and desserts that are just too tempting, give them to your guests to take home," says Janis Jibrin, M.S., R.D., author of *The Pescetarian Plan: The Vegetarian & Seafood Way to Lose Weight and Love Your Food.*

GF WANTS TO KNOW

What's the biggest diet mistake I can make when trying to maintain my ideal weight?

—Wanting to Learn, 38, Georgetown, MA

Dear GF,

Waiting until you're hungry to eat. And we don't mean *too* hungry. That's just an invitation to allow cravings to get in the way. Here's the GF rule of thumb: If you're going to have three or more hours between meals, work in a little low-calorie snack, so you don't end up at your next meal with a growler in your stomach. For more tips, see page 75 in Chapter 3.

MOVE THEM OUT OF SIGHT. Wrap and put leftovers away as soon as the partygoers leave so you aren't tempted to nibble as you clean up in the kitchen. Store particularly tempting goodies (like candy and packaged treats) in a tin on a high shelf in a cabinet so they're out of reach.

ICE IT. Pick up some small plastic containers when you're food shopping so you can freeze leftovers in reasonable portions, suggests Bonci. This offers a one-two punch: It curbs temptation (you can't open the fridge and indulge) *and* lengthens the life of your leftovers. Basically, any dish that doesn't contain raw vegetables will freeze well. Just make sure to pop the food in as soon as possible (don't refrigerate it for a day or two first) to prevent bacteria growth.

Watch out for ▸ A Bounty of Food at Holiday Parties

When you're hosting, you tend not to eat while the party is in full swing since you're busy making sure all of your guests are happy and well taken care of. But when you're a guest, celebrations can feel like an obstacle course: the buffet table, the bar, the passed hors d'oeuvres, the dessert table. Use these simple steps to navigate all the calorie and fat traps with ease.

SAVE YOUR APPETITE. "Try going to the party a little hungry, but not ravenous—just as you would feel when you sit down to any other meal," says Jabrin. "If it's an evening event, eat balanced meals throughout the day, but skip snacks and treats to leave some calories for later. If it's an afternoon party, eat your usual breakfast, and if you're hungry an hour or so beforehand, have a small snack (around 200 calories), like a medium sliced apple with a tablespoon of peanut butter."

SURVEY WHAT'S AVAILABLE. Take a look at *all* the appetizers before you start sampling, and if you know the host well enough, ask what she's serving as a main course. That way, you can choose a

GF WANTS TO KNOW

How can I survive a Super Bowl Party without a calorie hangover?

Party Girl in Milwaukee, WI

Dear GF,

Just like any holiday party, start with rule number one: Don't arrive hungry. Eat a filling breakfast and have a light meal a few hours before kickoff. It might seem like a good idea to save up your calories for the party, but in your hungry daze, you're more than likely to make bad food choices. Also, keep the alcohol tab low. Liquid calories add up quickly, and after a few drinks, you may have less self-control around the chicken wings and ribs. Fill your plate with all the good stuff you can find—anything green and vegetable. If you must, take a sampling of the bad stuff you just can't resist. One night isn't going to kill your diet, but remember, you must get back on track in the A.M.

It's the quintessential cocktail party star (except for the booze), and for good reason: Shrimp cocktail is scrumptious—and proof that the best food can have the *fewest* calories. Four large shrimp clock in at around 40 calories and the two tablespoons of cocktail sauce to turn it up a notch is only 40 calories. Double up and make a beeline straight to the crudités to load up on veggies, and you don't need dinner!

few foods you'd like to splurge on. If it's buffet-style, divide your plate and fill half with veggies. The other half should be a carb (brown rice, potatoes, whole-grain bread) and a protein. If there's a fatty food you really like, such as sausage, take just a taste, Jibrin suggests.

BE AWARE OF LITTLE BITES. They may look harmless, but mini appetizers often contain about 100 calories a pop and can easily add up without filling you up. "You eat them quickly, they're hard to keep track of, and they're not all that satisfying," says Jibrin. If you're splurging on the main course, choose lighter appetizers, such as sliced vegetables with dip—but keep it to a handful of veggies, since a tablespoon of dip is about 100 calories.

Watch out for ▸ Holiday Drinks

A five-ounce glass of eggnog or hot-buttered rum can cost you 400 calories and 20 grams of fat. It's like drinking a second lunch! If you just can't resist, take yours in a smaller cup or serving (cut it in half), and sip *slowly*. Or, whip up your own. Our girl-friendly bartender came up with this version with 105 calories (without the rum) and two grams of fat per serving. Like eggnog, you make it for a group.

Lighter Eggnog

MAKES 6½ CUPS OR 13 SERVINGS

3 lg. eggs

3 lg. egg whites

5½ c. low-fat milk

½ c. sugar

2 Tbsp. cornstarch

Salt

2 Tbsp. vanilla

½ tsp. plus a dash nutmeg

⅓ c. Jamaican rum
(optional)

1. In bowl, with whisk, beat eggs and egg whites until blended; set aside. In heavy 4-qt. saucepan, with heat-safe spatula, mix 4 c. milk with sugar, cornstarch and ¼ tsp. salt. Cook on medium-high until mixture boils and thickens slightly, stirring constantly. Boil 1 min. Remove saucepan from heat.

2. Gradually whisk ½ c. simmering milk mixture into eggs; pour egg mixture back into milk in saucepan, whisking constantly, to make custard.

3. Pour custard into large bowl; stir in vanilla, nutmeg, rum, if using, and remaining 1½ c. milk. Cover and refrigerate until well chilled, at least 6 hrs. or up to 2 days. Sprinkle eggnog with nutmeg to serve.

Watch out for ▸ Dessert Goodies Galore

Friends, neighbors, coworkers, your second cousin once removed—everyone's bearing treats this time of year. You need a plan of action to deal with the nonstop storm of tantalizing sweets:

THINK BEFORE YOU EAT. It's tempting to taste everything that comes your way, but pausing and asking yourself, *Do I really want to eat this? Do I like it enough that the calories are worth spending?*

It's not just winter holiday feasting that can trip you up—the calories at a summer barbecue can add up. We quizzed Becky Hand, registered dietitian and coauthor of *The Spark Solution*, about how she navigates the summer holiday spreads from Memorial Day through Labor Day.

For starters. "Chances are, there will be watermelon or corn on the cob—it's good to go for fresh produce first to fill up. Plus, they're in season and delicious!"

Burger or hot dog? "Burger. It may have about 215 calories—compared with 140 in a hot dog—but it has 22 grams of protein versus five, so it keeps you full longer, and there's also less sodium and fewer additives."

Potato salad or cole slaw: "Slaw. It could still be high in fat if it's made with mayo, but the carrots and cabbage have fiber and vitamins A and C. Limit yourself to a half cup."

can help stop you from mindlessly munching and racking up the calories.

SET UP A SCHEDULE. At home, pick one time of day (say, your 3 o'clock snack or a dessert) and what you're going to splurge on.

ASSIGN EACH COWORKER A WEEK TO BRING IN ONE TREAT. This will help control the onslaught at the office. You can also organize a healthy snack list and have coworkers bring in a nutritious option each day—for example, a crudités or fruit platter.

Oops! I Overdid It
Now what?!

Rule *numero uno*: Don't be too hard on yourself. "Your body regulates itself, so your metabolism speeds up a little when you eat more," says Janis Jibrin, M.S., R.D. You'd need to ingest about 5,000 calories in a single day to immediately gain a permanent pound.

Most day-after scale increases are temporary bloating. "The real trouble starts when a single day turns into weeks of overdoing it," she says. Black Friday is not the day to say, *I blew it. I'll just enjoy the holidays and get back to it again January 1.* This is what really leads to trouble and gets you into yo-yo dieting. So regroup!

Start your "fix" by steering clear of high-sodium foods, drink plenty of water and get back on track by following this easy morning-after plan:

TAKE A LONG WALK. Get out for at least a 30-minute walk first thing the morning after. This will help jump-start your metabolism and put you in a healthy-eating mind-set for the day.

FILL UP ON FIBER. Include at least one high-fiber food at each meal to help satisfy you for fewer calories—aim for an extra five grams of fiber that day by zeroing in on whole grains, fruits and vegetables. However, stay away from foods that cause gas and bloating, such as brussels sprouts and other cabbages, beans, lentils and turnips.

CUT BACK A LITTLE MORE. Whatever number of calories you were eating before the big goof-up, trim it back more severely for a few days. For example, if your goal is 1,600 calories a day, eat 1,400 for the next few days until the scale gets back to where you left off.

However, don't do it by skipping meals. Also, avoid indulgences like desserts and alcohol.

EAT SOME YOGURT. A few studies suggest that the good bacteria, or probiotics, in yogurt can help with digestion and ease bloating. Have plain low-fat yogurt to keep calories in check. To boost flavor, add a sprinkle of cinnamon or a small drizzle of honey.

GF Action Plan

All your hard effort to lose weight won't work if you go back to your bad habits around food. A maintenance program means learning to train your brain to change your behavior around food. *All* the tips in this chapter are worth adopting—they've been scientifically proven to work. But don't try to take them all on at once. Instead:

START A FOOD DIARY: If you haven't yet started recording your calories, do so now and add any thoughts or emotions that will help you tap into the source of your eating habits. (See Chapter 3 for more on food diaries.)

CREATE YOUR GROCERY SHOPPING STRATEGY: Do what works for you, whether it's the idea of cutting the shopping cart in half, finding new Mediterranean foods each week or weaning yourself away from the old favorites that you need to cut back on.

HAVE A HOLIDAY PARTY PLAN: Prepare yourself for these occasions when your guard can fall—what will you do before you reach for that extra glass of wine or helping of food?

PREPARE YOUR SNACK STASH: Always keep some healthy portable snacks in your handbag or briefcase so you don't get caught in the hunger trap.

As you look back on all the strategies in this chapter, pick the ones that resonate most with you and practice, practice, practice. Keep at it, and everything eventually will click.

Exercise:
The Other Half
Of Weight Loss

6

NO GYM? NO TRAINER? NO TIME? That pretty much sums up the lives of a lot of girlfriends we know and talk to. So let's be real: The best exercise for you is the one you'll actually do. And here's the deal: You can choose the way you want to sweat—be it walking, jogging, biking, even in-line skating—as long as you do it at least five days a week for at least 30 minutes. Studies show that's the minimum requirement it takes to get in shape, help promote weight loss and reap heart-healthy benefits. We're talking 150 minutes—just 2½ hours—a week. You can even do it in short spurts of 10 minutes and still get the same results. Combine it with the Mediterranean-style eating plan and the change-your-attitude-about-food strategies that make up The Girlfriends Diet, and you should be on your way to gradual and permanent weight loss, just like all the women you're reading about in these pages. You *will* see results. One yearlong study found that women who changed their diet *and* exercised lost 10.8% of their body weight, compared with a loss of 8.5% for those who tried through diet alone—a difference scientists note as "significant."

There isn't one person you've read about in this book who didn't achieve weight loss without fitting activity into her life. This doesn't mean you have to turn yourself into a marathoner like 105-pound-loser Jackie Freitag, or become an exercise guru to others, like Christi Borchers, who fell in love with Zumba and danced off 80 pounds. Stephanie Gee, a physician who dropped 40 excess pounds, found life to be less hectic when she stopped being maniacal about exercise. "I don't need to try to run marathons anymore. It took an injury for me to figure that out."

GF STAY SLIM SECRET

"Choose a diet and an exercise routine that fit your personality. I'd die from loneliness on a treadmill. But Zumba classes are like a party!"
— *Lauren McGoldrick,* Good Housekeeping *reader,*
Brooklyn, NY

All the women in this book discovered, as you will, that "*d-i-e-t*" is just another four-letter word. What it really takes to achieve the body you want is *change*—a lifestyle adjustment that focuses on healthy eating *and* being active. But intuitively you already know this, right? So let's make it happen. And guess what? You don't even have to step foot in a gym.

"Fitness *needs* to be part of your life," says Jillian Michaels, one of America's best-known personal trainers, frequently seen on *The Biggest Loser*. "But as long as you're getting your exercise somehow, it doesn't matter whether you're doing it in a gym or sweating it out alone or with a buddy in your backyard."

Thousands of older people in the Mediterranean regions who became the subject of scientific study because of their robust health and sleek bodies have never even seen the inside of a gym. If you asked them what they do for exercise, they'd tell you "nothing." That's because they don't think of their active lifestyle as "exercise." To them, it's just a natural part of living. They spend every day in almost constant motion. They wouldn't dream of getting in the car to drive a half mile to the grocery store. They walk or ride a bike—and they do it every day. They plant and harvest their own vegetables, knead their daily bread, pick apples from trees and berries from bushes, and work in the fields. And they walk, walk, walk—often up and down hills scores of times a day—to do chores and visit friends.

These are the people who have proved to the world that being active is not just about exercise. More important, it's about health. Regular exercise can help reduce your risk of just about *everything*, namely chronic conditions such as heart disease, cancer and diabetes. Exercise also triggers positive changes in your brain, including forging new connections between nerve cells, increasing blood flow and even creating new brain cells—all of which help strengthen your memory and problem-solving skills. A brisk half-hour walk every day can also lower your chances of developing dementia. Best of all, it's never too late to make a difference. Research shows that even longtime couch potatoes who start a regular exercise program can

Another Reason to Exercise

Always got food on the brain? There's a way to get it off the brain: Exercise.

Researchers at Brigham Young University found that women who trotted on a treadmill for 35 minutes in the morning were less excited by images of food (as assessed by an electroencephalogram) than those who simply rolled out of bed and started their day. Bonus: They were more active for the rest of the day, too.

experience positive changes in brain function almost immediately.

"Think about activity as a piggy bank," says Pamela Peeke, M.D., author of *Body for Life for Women*. "It's not about a gym, but if that's your thing, more power to you. However, ten minutes here and five minutes there toward that 30-minutes-a-day goal counts. So does an intense game of Wii bowling, and so does tossing a Frisbee around in the backyard. A 10-minute walk after each meal or a 15-minute stroll with your dog before and after work will do it for you, too. Simply getting up and moving around—whether it's from your desk at work during the day or while watching TV—immediately kicks your metabolism into gear."

Your Girlfriends Diet Club will no doubt talk plenty about exercise. You'll hear all about the desire to exercise and all the excuses why there's no time to do it. Truth be known, the biggest deterrent to exercise for most women has nothing to do with lack of energy; it's finding the motivation to make nonnegotiable time. That's where your diet club or diet buddies can come in—big-time. "To get yourself moving, recruit friends to work out with you, which builds a support system and holds you accountable when you'd rather park your butt on the couch," says Michaels. "There's no way I'd get out to the park for a 6 A.M. workout if I weren't picking up my neighbor down the block on the way," reports Jane von Mehren of Brooklyn, NY, of the boot camp sessions she and her neighbor take in the spring, summer and fall. So don't sit around talking about how to fit exercise into your life, walk around together and talk about it. You'll already be started!

A Girlfriends Diet Club is the perfect venue for group exercise. Incorporate activity into your planned weekly sessions. For example, do a walkabout to discuss your progress instead of sitting around a table or lounging in a living room. End the session with some yoga moves. Ask a different member each week to introduce a toning or

Working out with a group of friends does more than burn calories and make time fly. You'll definitely get fit, according to the results of 19 studies that followed group walking programs. There are also these tangible benefits:

Group workouts will make you happier: Any form of exercise will improve your mood, but group workouts boost endorphins even more than solo sessions, according to a University of Oxford study.

Team exercise will feel easier: Researchers who tracked people exercising alone or as a team found that when they were in a group, each person's pain threshold went up. Fist bump!

Outdoor exercise will chill you out: Exercising in a natural setting is more enjoyable—and may also be more motivating. It's not just the surroundings that give the lift, say British researchers. It's also the color green itself. When cyclists pedaled while watching unaltered videos of a woodsy environment, they felt happier and less fatigued than when they viewed the same scenery in black-and-white or filtered, in red. Such positive emotions probably make it easier to work out more often and for longer, says Dominic Micklewright, Ph.D., of the University of Essex.

flexibility exercise you all can practice during the week, the same way you would recommend what to read at a book club.

Get Your Body in Motion

Even though a tough workout can make us hungry, research has found that low-intensity exercise—the kind we are mostly recommending in this chapter—results in an energy deficit. In one study, women burned an average of about 177 more calories than they ate on their workout days. If you do low-intensity exercise five times a week, that's equal to a loss of 13 pounds in one year. How's that for incentive!

The workouts you'll find on the following pages are all professionally developed routines designed for women with too much on their plates—figuratively speaking, of course. Walking is the one thing we all can do, so consider it your *minimum* goal. You'll also find suggestions for cardio, which is important to your overall fitness and health; and some toning exercises, which will tighten muscles and help you maintain strength and stability as you get older. And don't overlook yoga. Explore this ages-old practice that benefits mind, body and spirit. It's an ideal and relaxing form of exercise that might appeal to your Girlfriends Diet Club as a group activity. Or just take it up on your own.

Whatever you decide, work your exercise goal around getting more movement in your daily life. The more active you are throughout the day, the more calories you'll burn. But there's more to it than just burning off calories. After reviewing studies on exercise and eating habits, Harvard University researchers came to the conclusion that activity induces positive changes in the area of the brain that governs willpower. You'll find it a lot easier to ignore the hors d'oeuvres tray as it passes by, or to say no to dessert when you're out

She did it!

ABBIE KRANTZ
AGE **37**
LOST **16 POUNDS!**

HERE'S HOW: "I'd said that I wanted to lose weight in the past, but I would never follow through. This time, when I started to exercise, everything clicked. My husband could see the transformation—not just physically, but emotionally—and he was very supportive, offering to watch the kids so I could work out. Before, I was always thinking about my muffin top and tugging at my clothes to hide my tummy. It's great not to be so self-conscious anymore."

AMANZING! MAKEOVER!

Christi Borchers
"I lost 80 pounds—and finally found the job I love."

I NOW KNOW WHY I spent my 30s weighing more than 200 pounds. There was my health: I grew up having asthma, which turned me off sports, and then I was diagnosed with a thyroid condition that made losing weight difficult. There was also my lifestyle: I married a Navy guy, and we were always moving—12 times in 18 years—which made it hard to stick to healthy routines.

When our son, Jackson, was born in 2001, I felt lonely caring for him. In each new city, I'd get a little more depressed, a little heavier and a little more ashamed. I would snack all day, especially on anything cheesy. Then I'd have a big dinner with my husband to hide from him how much I'd eaten all day.

My low point came in 2005 when we moved to Japan. We were living in

this amazing place, but at 5'5" and 253 pounds, I had such bad arthritis in my knee I had to walk with a cane.

Two years later when we moved back to the United States, to Virginia, I was able to lose 15 pounds, but things really didn't turn around for another two years when I reconnected with my old friend Michelle. We decided we'd team up to lose weight and joined the Y. We really needed each other to stay motivated because it was so hard just going to the gym. We kept hearing music coming from the Zumba class and we'd peek in, but we were too intimidated to go in. I loved the party vibe of Zumba, but it took awhile for us to work up the nerve to try it, and when we finally did, we hid in the back. I may be from Nebraska farm country, but that Latin

beat got me instantly *hooked*!

At first our goal was just to get through a class. My knee prevented me from jumping and my weight made me self-conscious, but the instructor's encouragement kept me going. In January 2010, I committed to two classes a week. It was a bumpy ride: I had been unhappy about my body for so long, and you can't reverse those feelings overnight. But the weight started falling off.

More important, Zumba totally changed my view of exercise. I am totally hooked on group exercise. A treadmill won't smile at you or push you to achieve your goals like a great teacher or friend will. Of course, I changed how I ate, too. Because of all my years of yo-yo dieting, I hated the "D" word, but I made gradual changes, like cutting back on sugar and other refined carbs. My husband totally supported my efforts—I discovered you can't achieve something this big without the support of those you care about along the way. We grill together and eat lots of vegetables. But if I want a piece of cheesecake, I have one.

We live in Colorado now, and today my life is totally changed. I don't just take Zumba classes, I *teach* them. And I tell my story to my students and hope it will inspire them. I got down to a healthy weight of 158 pounds that I've been able to maintain. My cholesterol levels and blood pressure aren't high anymore, my thyroid is more regulated, and my knee is much better. Shopping for clothing is an amazing experience for me now. I still reach for larger sizes when I get into stores, then have to work my way down.

The best thing, though, is that Michelle and I are

"A treadmill won't smile at you or push you to achieve your goals like a great teacher or friend will."

still together supporting each other. Even though we are states apart, we talk almost every day— usually about Zumba. She's certified to teach it, too, and we plan to get together at a Zumba conference in San Diego in a few months. We're also meeting up soon for a girlfriends' weekend in Nashville—and I'll have my playlist with me, so I can lead a class for my friends in the hotel.

You might say I'm exercise-dependent now. I lead a class every day and take at least another three classes in a group. Still, keeping a positive body image can be a struggle. On tougher days, I remind myself that it's my job to be upbeat. If necessary, I assume my alter ego: Sparkle pants, the nickname my Zumba girlfriends gave me. I weigh myself weekly, but the scale no longer rules my emotions. The endorphins I get from exercise are my go-to solution. They last much longer than a doughnut!

When it comes to achieving a goal and maintaining the weight that you've lost, I always remind myself that it's about progress, not perfection. No matter how slowly you go, you're still lapping everyone who's sitting on the couch!

to dinner, or to skip that second helping of sweet potato pie at Thanksgiving. And don't forget the most *important* reason: Dozens of studies show that active people are healthier, happier and live longer than slouch potatoes.

You know the deal: Never ride when you can walk, take the stairs instead of the elevator, walk the perimeter of the supermarket before you start to shop, park as far away as possible from the door at the mall, walk to deliver a message to a coworker instead of zipping off an e-mail—and so on! To keep track of your movement, attach a pedometer to your belt. It's a great way to get you stepping more and keep you motivated. The common goal recommended by experts is to move enough during the day to equal 10,000 steps—about five miles. Here's the sneaky-cool thing: Unless you're a nurse or a waitress who walks the floor all day, it's pretty hard to get in 10,000 steps a day without fitting in at least a 30-minute walk. So tie on those sneakers, and let's move.

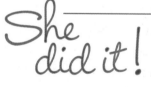

HEATHER WELLS
AGE **42**
LOST **6 POUNDS!**

HERE'S HOW: "I often look back at a picture of me from my honeymoon in a T-shirt and cargos. I wasn't in perfect shape; I wasn't even at a perfect weight—whatever 'perfect' means, anyway—but I was healthy and I felt good. That's what I wanted to return to. My husband and I started to eat better after having a child—less junk, more fruits and vegetables. But I still got in trouble with too-big portions. Cutting back helped a lot.

"I knew I needed to start working out, so I walked and did the Wii Fit at home. But my body didn't begin to change until I upped the intensity. Once I started taking spin classes and following the workout on Jillian Michaels's *30 Day Shred* DVD, I started to see a difference. I lost four inches off my waist and hips, and 2½ inches off my thighs. I'm fitting into clothes that are three sizes smaller, and I'm still going. I never thought I'd say this, but if I skip a workout, I miss it!"

Walk, Walk, Walk

Walking just sounds too easy to be *real* exercise, but it really is. So, repeat after us: *There is no excuse not to walk!*

"Walking is a great way to burn calories and get in shape," says Ramona Braganza, Hollywood's go-to trainer. "I tell my clients, walk as if you're late for an appointment—briskly. Getting your heart rate up is key to improving your cardiovascular fitness. To make it more intense, you could also carry a water bottle in each hand. The added stress resistance forces you to use every muscle in your legs, back and core. Aim for 10,000 steps. If you wear a pedometer, you'll see how quickly those steps add up just by sneaking in short walks."

If you do nothing but walk, you should still lose weight, says Braganza. "If you weigh 180 pounds, you'll burn 100 calories in a mile. If you weight 120 pounds, you'll burn 65. Do it consistently, and you'll change your weight, your body and your health."

Now, that's incentive!

Once you get comfortable walking and can go at a good clip for a nonstop 30 minutes, you can really stoke the burn with this ultimate walking routine developed by Michele Olson, Ph.D., certified strength and conditioning specialist and professor of exercise science at Auburn University at Montgomery. It incorporates Tabata bursts, which are short intervals of heart-pumping resistance moves that help you burn more calories. If you simply strolled for 30 minutes at a brisk pace, you'd burn about 170 calories, but with this easy plan, you'll torch 245. That's an extra 75 calories—gone!

> ### ▌ THE ULTIMATE WALKING WORKOUT
>
> **1.** Walk at a brisk pace for 13 minutes. As Braganza says, walk as if you're late for an appointment or trying to get to the gate of a boarding plane.
>
> **2.** Next, do this two-minute Tabata burst:

Squat Stand Stand with feet shoulder-width apart and arms bent in front of you. Your fists should be in line with your shoulders. Squat down like you're sitting in a chair, then stand back up on your tiptoes and extend your arms straight up over your head. Repeat this movement for 20 seconds, then rest for 10 seconds. Do one more set.

High-Knee Skip Mimic jumping rope as you lift your knees, one at a time, and twirl your arms for 20 seconds. Rest for 10 seconds, then do one more set.

3. Then walk at a brisk pace for 13 more minutes.

4. Finally, do this two-minute Tabata burst:

March and Lift March in place, raising your knees as high as possible, for 20 seconds. Rest for 10 seconds, then do one more set.

Mogul Jumps Stand with your feet together and your arms at your sides. Squat down and jump to one side, then back to the other side (as if you're jumping over a yardstick on the ground). Repeat this movement for 20 seconds. Rest for 10 seconds, then do one more set.

GF STAY SLIM SECRET
"When I really don't feel like exercising, I just put on some upbeat music and dance for half an hour."
—*Jamie Watson,* Good Housekeeping *reader, Wheat Ridge, CO*

Fix Your Form

You can reduce your risk of injury *and* increase your calorie burn by improving your walking form and stride, says Jessica Matthews, an exercise physiologist and spokesperson for the American Council on Exercise. Here is what she recommends:

HEAD Look up. Try to focus about 10 feet to 20 feet in front of you, which will naturally help your head stay where it should be—*not* hunched forward.

SHOULDERS Press both your shoulders down so they're away from your ears.

ARMS Bend your elbows at 90 degrees and keep them close to your sides. Make a loose fist with your hands. Imagine that you're holding something small, like a potato chip. Gripping too tightly can cause numbness in hands and fingers.

HIPS Try to lead with your hips as you walk, rather than with your upper body.

FEET Think of each step as a roll: Start with the heel, then roll through the midfoot and push off with the toes. Learning to roll as you stride, instead of landing flat-footed, will help prevent pain in your shins and knees.

SHOES Walking shoes should have flexible soles to allow your feet to move naturally. One easy way to make sure a pair passes the test: Fold a shoe in half, then twist it side to side. If the soles of the shoes are too stiff and don't bend at all, don't buy them.

> **CELEB GF ADVICE**
> *When I go offtrack occasionally, I do a 'shape-up week' to focus myself again. I work out every day and eat super-clean."*
> —Alison Sweeney, host of The Biggest Loser

Cardio: The Fat-Burning Workout

If this is the year you really want to get rid of the pouch hanging over your jeans, then you need to get into cardio, the type of exercise that gets your heart rate up and gets you huffing and puffing. "It is the key to burning belly fat," says celebrity trainer Holly Perkins.

Duke University researchers demonstrated this when they had a group of overweight women do 45 minutes of either aerobic or resistance training three times a week. The cardio group lost the most weight and fat. And while a third group that did both workouts also lost more pounds and more fat than the women who did only resistance training, it was not significantly greater than what the aerobic-only exercisers lost—and they had to log twice as much time!

 GF GET MOVING SECRET "My very crazy and embarrassing playlist keeps my workout fun. I've been caught doing some interesting dance moves with my arms while running."

—Jacqui Goldberg O'Connell,
Good Housekeeping *reader, Pensacola, FL*

High-intensity workouts "have been proven to burn more calories both during and after your exercise," Perkins says. Here's how it goes: Four days a week for 35 to 40 minutes, do any sweat-inducing exercise you like, such as jogging, biking, rowing, swimming or the elliptical trainer. On two of those days, do the Steady-Pace Workout. On the other two days, do the Interval Workout.

▸ **STEADY-PACE WORKOUT**

Warm up by exercising gently for five minutes, then increase the intensity until you've exercised at what feels like a 7 on a scale of 1 to 10, with 10 being really tough. Try to stay at this intensity for 35 minutes, then cool down for five minutes.

▸ **INTERVAL WORKOUT**

Warm up gently for five minutes. Then sprint, amping up the intensity, for two minutes (you'll want to eventually aim for what feels like a 9 on that scale of 1 to 10. Then slow down and go easy for two minutes. Repeat this cycle for a total of 25 minutes, then cool down for five minutes.

Dear GF,

Here's the GF game plan: Instead of running until you're so pooped you stop—that only gets you in the habit of quitting—mix short intervals of running with walking three times a week to build stamina. Warm up with a five-minute walk, then alternate 30 seconds of jogging with 30 seconds of walking for a mile and a half. Add 30 seconds to the run portions and a half mile to your distance each week. In a month, you'll be up to three miles, jogging most of the time. Now you're ready to run a 5K race and with the excitement of race day, and you'll fly through 3.1 miles!

If working out with an app appeals to you, here's another option: Couch-to-5K, a program for beginners.

"Steady-pace workouts are easier to maintain for longer periods of time so you can tap into your fat-burning zone," Perkins says. "They'll also improve your aerobic fitness—and help clear your head. The short blasts of the interval workouts allow you to work out harder and raise your heart rate, which increases your metabolism for three or four hours post exercise."

You're still burning calories after you stop—how cool is that!

Ab-Fab Workouts

In anticipation of rocking your favorite little black dress as you walk the weight off, we asked three trainers to the stars for their best get-results flat-abs routines:

Easy

Brooke Siler, a celebrity Pilates instructor and owner of re:AB in New York City, teaches this core-strengthening move to all of her students. Do it daily or at least five times a week.

▶ CORE STRENGTHENER

1. Lie on your back with your knees bent at a right angle and your arms alongside you. Then lift your arms and pump them up and down, keeping them straight. Meanwhile, inhale for five counts and exhale for five counts, building up to 100 counts.

2. For more of a challenge, do the move with your head off the floor: Bring your head up to look at your belly button, making sure you're pulling up without straining your neck.

She did it!

SHYNO CHACKO PANDEYA
AGE **40**

"After my second child, my stomach never returned to normal—I used all my energy up just being a mom. Then, when it was time to go back to work, I thought, *Oh, my god, people are going to think I made this up—that I hadn't actually given birth!* I still had to wear my maternity pants. Every other part of my body was going back to my pre-baby shape, but there was all this stuff just sitting on my tummy, all this muffin top. I knew I had to get serious about exercise or I'd never get out of those pants. I figured out a workout that

"I lost 40 pounds and four inches off my belly."

was easy to incorporate into my life. I kept a yoga mat at work, and I'd shut my office door and do ab-toning exercises. As for the cardio, it's been a matter of slipping it in where I can. I'll put the kids in a double stroller and head to the park for speed walking. I'm down to a size 8 from a size 12, and my muffin top is gone."

Dear GF,

Sorry, girlfriend, we're going to say what you probably *don't* want to hear: The unfortunate truth is, most of us don't exercise enough to justify extra calories, especially when we're trying to lose weight. However, if you've restricted your calories enough that you're steadily losing weight, you can probably add an extra 100 calories to your day's total, but only on days when you work out for *at least* an hour. And you can add another 100 for every hour after that. Remember, you don't have to do it all in an hour or two. If, say, you take two brisk 30-minute walks and spend an hour in hot yoga, you should be able to add around 150 calories or so without sabotaging your weight-loss efforts.

Keep in mind, though, that every body is different and your rate of weight loss depends on your individual metabolism. In the end, what the scale is telling you should be your guide. And here's a bonus tip: To help maintain your stamina, take those extra calories in protein at breakfast—a scoop of cottage cheese or an egg, perhaps—or eat an extra snack of almonds or string cheese.

Not Too Hard

Celebrity trainer Holly Perkins designed this crunch-free workout to uncover and tone your abs. "These exercises work the entire core from front to back, which not only improves posture and prevents injury, but also creates a lean, tight-looking torso," Perkins says. Do the routine three times a week—you should be able to knock it back in less than 15 minutes—and see results in about three months. You'll need a pair of two-pound weights or a two-pound soft exercise ball.

STANDING OVERHEAD PRESS

Stand with your feet shoulder-width apart, holding a weighted ball or dumbbell with both hands. Pull your abs in tight, then lift your arms straight overhead, actively reaching up as high as you can for 10 counts. Lower your arms, and repeat five times.

LEG SWAP

Lie on your back with your knees bent, feet flat on the floor, holding the ball. Press the ball or a weight with your hands to the ceiling while pulling your abs in. Slowly lift your right leg, keeping your knee bent, until your leg is perpendicular to your body. Keeping your abs tight, lower your right foot to the floor as you simultaneously lift your left leg. Do two sets of 10 reps.

LYING BALL EXTEND

Lie on your back with your knees bent, feet flat on the floor, holding a weight with both hands. Raise your arms overhead until the weight rests on the ground. Tighten your abs and hold for one count; then, on an exhale, bring your chin toward your chest and curl your shoulders off the floor, lifting your arms several inches while keeping your elbows next to your ears. Hold for two counts, then release. Do two sets of 10 reps.

BALL BRIDGE

Lie on your back, knees bent, feet flat on the floor. Place the ball or a weight between your inner thighs. Pull your abs in tight, then press your heels into the floor to lift your pelvis, squeezing your thighs together. Hold for 10 counts, then lower. Repeat five times.

LYING OVERHEAD PRESS

Lie on your back, knees bent, feet flat on the floor, holding a weight at your chest with both hands. Tighten your abs, bring your chin toward your chest, and curl your shoulders off the floor. Push the weight overhead and back, so your elbows are next to your ears. Bring the weight back to your chest, then lower your head and shoulders back down. Do two sets of 10 reps.

▶ **ELBOW PLANK**

Kneel on the floor and place the ball or a weight between your thighs. Place your forearms on the floor, elbows directly under your shoulders. Pull your abs in tight and stretch both feet out behind you. Squeeze the ball and hold this pose for 20 seconds. Do three reps.

"My favorite music—high-energy '80s tunes—motivates me when I really don't want to exercise."

—*Sue Macaluso Lail,* Good Housekeeping *reader, Cape Vincent, NY*

Harder

We asked trainer Harley Pasternak how he's helped Lady Gaga, Katy Perry and Jennifer Hudson tone their abs. "You've got to do all three of these moves if you want to look great from every angle," he insists. Do three sets of 20 for each, three times a week—not just until you get to the abs you want, but to keep them toned. You'll need a medicine ball, or the equivalent, and a set of hand weights.

⊰ Bethenny's Flat-Belly Move ⊱

Yoga instructor Kristin McGee created this flat-belly move for Bethenny Frankel's DVD *Body by Bethenny*:

Sit on the floor with your legs straight, hands on the floor just behind your hips for support. With your back straight, lean back to a 45-degree angle, then bend your knees and lift your legs so your calves are parallel to the floor. Bring your arms to your sides in front of you at shoulder level. This is the starting position. Pull your belly in and slowly lean farther back, until your shoulder blades are a few inches from the floor. Hold for five counts, and return to the start. Repeat five times.

▶ DOUBLE CRUNCH

Lie on your back, hands behind your head, knees bent and feet flat on the floor. As you bring your chest up (like in a regular crunch), lift your knees up and touch your elbows to them.

▶ TRUNK TWIST

Sit on the floor with your knees bent, feet on the floor in front of you. Look straight ahead and lean back 30 degrees. Holding a medicine ball (or a watermelon), slowly rotate your upper body to the left, then to the right.

▶ SIDE BEND

Stand upright with an 8- to 10-pound dumbbell in your right hand hanging down at your side and your left hand against your left temple (as if you're saluting). Slowly slide the dumbbell down your right side as you lengthen your left arm and stretch it over toward the right. Slide the dumbbell back up as you return your left arm to its original position. Repeat on the other side.

Butt-Toning Routines

For a butt that does a pencil skirt justice, try one of these routines:

Really Easy

Here are two moves you can do without ever leaving your chair. Do each one 10 times, then repeat both moves:

▶ HEEL PRESS

FIRMS: Thighs, glutes and hamstrings
Sit on the edge of your chair with your knees bent. Keeping your feet flat, press your heels into the floor, hold for a few seconds, then release.

▶ CROSS ANKLE

FIRMS: Outer thighs and glutes
Sit up straight and cross your right ankle over your left, pressing the outside edges of your feet together. Hold for a few seconds, then relax.

Kim K's Favorite Butt Burner

This side lunge how-to is courtesy of Kim Kardashian's trainer Gunnar Peterson. It takes a little effort, so you'll feel the burn.

1. Stand with your feet hip-width apart, holding a light dumbbell or water bottle in each hand.

2. Take a big step out to the side with your left foot and lower into a squat, bending your left knee but keeping your right leg straight. Tap the weights to the floor, one on either side of your left foot.

3. Straighten up and step back to the starting position, then switch sides and repeat. That's one rep; do two sets of 20 reps.

Easy

We all have those days when we want to lie down and never get up. Put them to work for you with this move from Tracey Mallett, creator of the Booty Barre workout. Try it anytime you're just lying around, and feel the backside and leg toning.

> **BOAT POSE**
> Lie facedown on a rug, with your legs and arms extended, palms on the floor. Simultaneously lift your right arm and left leg six to eight inches off the floor. Then quickly switch arms and legs, lifting your left arm and right leg. Alternate 15 times. Rest, then do another 15.

Hard

This routine, courtesy of New York City trainer Liz DiAlto of Willspace, is definitely not for the faint of exercise. It is a CliffsNotes version of her booty-focused class, As*pire. Do it three times a week, and she says you'll see results in three weeks.

CARDIO ▸ 10 MINUTES

Run or power walk on an inclined treadmill or cycle with resistance.

SIDE LUNGE ▸ 1 MINUTE

Stand straight, abs tight, toes forward, left foot planted on the ground, right foot on a folded towel. Now sit back into your left butt (like a squat) while sliding the right leg straight out to the side. Return to standing by engaging your inner thigh and sliding your right foot back. Continue for 30 seconds; switch legs.

GLUTE BRIDGE HAMSTRING CURL ▸ 30 SECONDS

Lie on your back, arms at your sides, legs straight out in front, toes up, heels pressed into a folded towel. Now lean into your shoulder blades as you squeeze your glutes and slide your heels toward your butt while lifting your hips up into a bridge. Hold for two counts; release; repeat.

JUMP SQUAT ▸ 30 SECONDS

Grasp each end of the towel and stretch your arms out in front of you, feet shoulder-width apart, core tight. Lower yourself as if you were sitting into a chair. Now lift your arms up as you jump up, landing back into a squat. Repeat.

REST ▸ 30 SECONDS

REPEAT LAST FOUR STEPS TWO MORE TIMES ▸ 5 MINUTES

REPEAT CARDIO ▸ 10 MINUTES

Beach Party Moves

Heading for the beach for a girlfriends' weekend or a vacation with the kids? A little sand under your toes (and your belly) can take your workout to the max—even without any added weights. Get out there with your buddies early in the morning. You'll likely discover you're not the only ones doing a beach party workout.

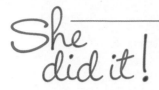
She did it!

SHNIEKA JOHNSON
AGE **30**

"In my 20s, before I had my son, I never had to worry much about my stomach. But after I had a baby, my weight fluctuated, and sometimes my belly protruded almost as far out as my breasts. I had all these cute dresses in my closet that were way too tight. In photos, I'd try to position myself a certain way to hide my belly. I thought, *How much longer can I suck it in?* I didn't think I had time to work out.

"I've now proved that 'I can't lose this tummy' was just a story I told myself. I figured out ways to make an exercise program work. I did belly exercises when my son was sleeping. I started using a stationary bike at home to get in my cardio when I couldn't make it to the gym. About four weeks in, I could actually feel the tightening in my core. When I noticed my pants fitting looser, that really motivated me. I formed a group in Google Plus and invited friends to join and cheer me on."

"My virtual friends kept me motivated."

This routine comes from Teddy Bass, who trains celebrities like Cameron Diaz on the California coast. Tackle these moves at least three or four times a week on your beach break. "The soft sand is gentler on the joints and offers more resistance," says Bass.

▶ **PLANK DROP**
TONES: Core, obliques, arms, chest, shoulders
Start as if you're about to do push-ups. Drop onto your right elbow, then onto your left elbow. Toes pushing into the sand and abs tight, push yourself back up—right arm first, then left—to your original position. Do five to 10 times; repeat, dropping onto your left elbow.

CRAB WALK

TONES: Triceps, glutes, back, calves, shoulders, posture

Sit on the sand, knees bent, palms down. Press up (like you're doing a reverse push-up), tightening your abs and butt. Starting with your left leg and right hand, followed by your right leg and left hand, walk backward—reaching as far behind you as possible—for one minute. Rest for a minute; repeat. Rest another minute; repeat.

JUMP SQUATS

TONES: Quads, glutes, hamstrings, calves, core

Squat as if you're about to sit into a chair—feet hip-width apart, arms by your hips. Now jump, arms shooting up into the air. As you come down, return to original "sitting" position.

Allover Toners

Here are a couple of allover toning exercises that are easy enough to fit in when you're just hanging out watching TV or preparing dinner.

Easy

This exercise, called a beginner's burpee, is a great multitasker, working your arms, shoulders, chest, back, core and lower body, says Leigh Crews, spokesperson for the American Council on Exercise and a certified personal trainer and fitness instructor. It goes from a push-up to a standing jump, and you can do it at the kitchen counter. Do two sets of 10.

GF GET MOVING SECRET

"I prepay for Zumba and yoga classes. Once I've spent my money, I'm more likely to stick with it."

—*Camille Linke,* Good Housekeeping *reader, Branford, CT*

Kelly Osbourne's Waist Whittler

Trainer Sarah Hagaman developed this waist-trimming exercise for Kelly Osbourne, who went on to lose 50 pounds during and after *Dancing with the Stars*. "Kelly's waistline was her weakest area in terms of strength and appearance, but she got dramatic results doing this core workout," says Hagaman. It incorporates a Bosu ball, which looks like half of a ball.

1. Rest the small of your back on a Bosu or stability ball, with knees bent and your arms out to the sides at shoulder level, in a "T."

2. Straighten your left leg, lift it off the ground, and twist to reach your right hand toward your left calf.

3. Switch sides. Lift your right leg and bring your left hand to your right calf. That's one rep. Do it 15 times.

BEGINNER'S BURPEE

1. Stand in front of a table or counter up to three feet high. Bend over and place your hands on the top of the ledge, then step your feet back one at a time so your torso forms a straight line. Do a push-up.

2. Walk your feet back in, stand up and raise your arms over your head.

3. To bump up the burn, add a jump when you return to standing, or use a lower surface, like a kitchen chair, for your push-up.

4. Do two sets of 10

Not Too Hard

Work your upper and lower body with this move from Jason Karp, Ph.D., coauthor of *Running for Women*. It calls for light hand weights, but two cans of beans (or soup, tomato sauce or artichokes) will work just as well.

1. Stand with your feet shoulder-width apart. Holding a dumbbell in each hand, lift your arms out to your sides and bend your elbows to 90-degree angles with your palms and arms facing forward.

2. Step forward with your right leg. Bend it until your thigh is parallel to the ground as you press the dumbbells over your head. Return to standing with feet shoulder-width apart, elbows to 90-degree angles; then repeat, stepping forward with your left leg. Continue, alternating sides, for 60 seconds.

GF GET MOVING SECRET

"Watching home improvement TV while I'm exercising ensures that I'll work out for as long as it takes to see the big reveal."
— *Stephanie Hanson,* Good Housekeeping *reader,*
Washington, DC

Harder

If you like to ski, this one's for you. It was designed by Stephanie Levinson, who created the Aspen Ascent class at Sports Club/LA. In addition to being an allover toner, it is designed to improve balance and strength, regardless of whether you'll be heading out to the snowy slopes.

▶ SWEEPING SQUAT

Stand with your feet hip-width apart, holding 5- to 8-pound dumbbells. Sit back into a low squat with your weight on your heels. Now sweep your arms to the sides, then stretch to the sky. Keep standing on your slightly bent right leg as you lift your left leg out to the side. Return to the original squat position, placing weights on floor. Repeat on the same side but without weights. Repeat all on right side. Do eight sets on each side.

Lie on your back with your head and neck two inches above the floor, hands behind your head, knees bent, feet flat on floor. Place paper plates (if you're on a carpet) or a towel (if you're on a wood floor) under your heels. Lift your chest up to your knees as you would in a crunch. Then, as your upper body returns to the ground, straighten your knees as your feet slide out. Return to the starting position and repeat.

Om, What's That You're Doing?

The slow and serene moves of yoga are well-known to help you shed stress, the number one reason why people give up on a diet. What is less commonly known is yoga's ability to help you shed pounds. Two new studies suggest that doing yoga can be effective in helping you lose weight, make you less likely to gain weight and give you a healthier body image. And it has nothing to do with the calories you're burning on the mat. Yoga enhances the connection between mind and body, making you less likely to overeat.

"When you're more in touch with your body, you're less likely to abuse it," says Deborah Patz Clarke, Psy.D., whose research found that people with binge-eating disorder were less likely to binge after

Turn on the Tube

You'll always have an exercise buddy on call when you log on to YouTube's BeFiT channel (youtube.com/befit), which offers free videos from fitness experts. New work-outs—from the likes of Jillian Michaels and Jane Fonda—are posted every weekday. Most of the routines are short—15 minutes or less—so you can easily squeeze one into your schedule.

doing 10 weeks of yoga. And you don't have to become a devotee to reap yoga's healthy-body benefits. In a study published in the *Journal of the American Dietetic Association*, women who practiced yoga only once a week ate more mindfully, meaning they were more aware of what they were eating, and how much—and were more likely to maintain a healthy weight.

While yoga videos can do the trick, study coauthor Celia Framson, R.D., recommends group classes for beginners. "Find an instructor you connect with," Framson says. "A good teacher can strengthen the mind-body connection."

ADVICE FROM A BESTIE

"Yes, yoga can help you slim down"

"I always remind friends that no one can tell you what will or won't work for you. Three years ago, when I wanted to slim down, no one suggested that I do yoga for exercise. But that's what I did. In the past, I didn't listen to my body. I'd get on the treadmill even though I had back pain because I thought it was what I was 'supposed' to do to lose weight, and I ended up herniating two disks. I tried Chrissy Carter's *Beginning Yoga* DVD to help with my recovery, and right away I knew it was the kind of workout my body needed. It strengthened my body, and it helped me really get in touch with myself. As a result, I began to feed myself differently, measuring my food and eating more fruits and veggies. That one decision to try yoga kick-started everything, and the weight came off."

—*Tricia Ostermann, 35, Brooklyn, NY, lost 60 pounds*

GF Action Plan

If you want to help speed up your weight loss, rev up your metabolism through exercise:

PURCHASE A PEDOMETER. Aim to log *at least* 10,000 steps a day.

You may need to work up to it, but just keep adding steps every day until you reach that goal. Remember, walking the dog, making the beds or pacing while you're on the phone all count!

FIND A TONING OR STRENGTH ROUTINE THAT WORKS FOR YOU. Toning exercises help you flatten your abs and tighten your butt. They also help build muscle, which helps keep your metabolism burning.

SCHEDULE A GROUP FITNESS CLASS or activity with your Girl-friends Diet Club or diet buddies. Working out in a group will keep you motivated.

* Order a copy of *The Girlfriends Diet* for your friend at goodhousekeeping.com/girlfriends.
* Share your success stories and get more dieting tips on our Facebook page at facebook.com/girlfriendsdiet.

chapter 7 The Girlfriends Diet Gets Social

A FEW YEARS BACK, a major household products company conducted a survey in which it asked women to rate their responsibilities by order of importance in their lives. The results?

1. Kids

2. Home

3. Job/career

4. Family pet(s)

5. Spouse

6. Yourself

You're probably laughing out loud right now over the pet-above-spouse revelation, but what's sobering about this true confession is the acknowledgment of where we see ourselves. Doctors say one of the biggest mistakes they see women make is putting themselves last on their list of to-dos. *Get mom to her doctor's appointment:*

Check! *Help the kids with their homework:* Check! *Beg the hub to get a physical:* Check! *Sneak in a trip to the gym:* Whoops—that one fell off the list. *Get back on the diet tomorrow:* That one never even made it on the list.

Even women who understand the importance of healthy eating and exercise are surprised to find out that putting themselves last in their list of obligations is a blueprint for stress and an *un*healthy lifestyle. We worry about everybody else eating right, but somehow we can't always make it work for ourselves. Then, one day the zipper doesn't make it all the way up and we're shopping for Spanx. We're left wondering how all that running around can possibly be *adding* weight instead of taking it off. Which is why The Girlfriends Diet's focus on creating a club or finding diet buddies to support your weight-loss journey is not just a fun idea, it is a sound, stress-relieving idea. An important, healthy idea. A let's-make-our-diet-fun idea.

Play More, Eat Less

We've all had those moments when we know we need a time-out from life for a little fun, or else we'll start acting *really* irrational—and it often happens around food. "As a society, we're so removed from the concept of adult fun that we don't even know what it is," says Brené Brown, Ph.D., a researcher and professor at the University of Houston and the author of *Daring Greatly*. "Yet there's a clear relationship between fun and how much joy and fulfillment people experience in their lives." In fact, when researchers followed the routines of more than 6,000 people, they found that fun deprivation can have consequences similar to sleep deprivation: Without it, our overall wellness and happiness, our creativity and relationships, and our willpower around food, all begin to droop. "It's a health issue, as important as exercise, eating right or taking vitamins," says Brown.

If we don't make time for fun, we miss out on a regular source of happiness. Getting together with your buddies—whether it be for a weekly happy hour or a weekend tennis match—boosts your mood because it forces the brain to relax. And when your mood is high, so is your willpower. It reinforces your goals for losing weight. "The mind at play is active and alert," says Peter Gray, a research professor of psychology at Boston College who studies the evolution of play. It doesn't have time to stew over the weeds in the garden or crave an ice cream cone. In fact, Tobin Quereau and Tom Zimmerman, coauthors of *The New Game Plan for Recovery*, believe that remembering to have fun is essential for people who tend to reach for outside fixes, such as food or alcohol, to escape life. Says

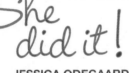

JESSICA ODEGAARD
AGE **25**
LOST **82 POUNDS!**

HERE'S HOW: "When my sister asked me to be maid of honor at her wedding, I was thrilled—but anxious. I thought, *I'm so fat, I'll wreck her photos.* I was in my early 20s and 213 pounds. I had been struggling with my weight since puberty and had gone on so many diets before, and I had failed so many times that I would be too embarrassed to tell anyone that I was trying again, so I'd end up just giving up. My sister's engagement was the breaking point for me— that and too many people saying, 'You have such a pretty face.' That meant, 'Why don't you lose weight?' So I signed up for a local group where people talk about their struggles and support each other. Clearly, dieting in secret wasn't working for me. The support of my family, boyfriend, and new friends blew me away. Everyone was totally behind my doing this for my health. It was hugely motivational.

"By my sister's wedding in May 2011, I was down 49 pounds. Two years later, I reached my goal of 131 pounds—down 82 pounds! Maintaining the loss as the weight was coming off has been a challenge, but exercising three times a week definitely helps. That and knowing that my healthy new weight is the way I want to live."

Quereau: "It can be hard to have fun when you're depressed, but it's just as hard to stay depressed when you're having fun."

So what does fun mean in the adult world? As the experts define it, it's something you do solely for enjoyment. It requires your mind and body to be wholly active—kind of like watching a thriller with a plot that fully engages you versus mindlessly clicking through Facebook.

Even if scheduling time to put yourself first sounds about as care-free as scheduling sex sounds romantic, you have to do it. "Considering how important it is, we should protect that time as fiercely as we do our doctor's appointments," says Brown. And, if you're too busy or "too old for that kind of stuff," remind yourself of this: The fun police exist only in our minds.

Girls Just Want to Have Fun

One of the reasons "going on a diet" works against us, especially when we do it alone, is because it gets us in the mind-set that the rest of life has to be put on hold. However, if you think of your "diet" as part of a healthy *lifestyle*, it puts you in a different state of mind. Letting loose can take you to a place of unexpected joy. Try it, and experience uplifting rewards.

Getting together with your diet buddies for fun can be anything you want it to be, but you'll get the most satisfaction out of it if you aim for something that keeps you and your girlfriends active. Make one meeting a month a Girls' Night Out or a Girls' Night In where you can meet and have fun over a cocktail and dinner—a perfect venue for learning how to eat out while losing weight. For your Girls' Night Out, there are strategies for how to eat at different kinds of restaurants without straying from your dietary goals, starting on page 200. For a Girls' Night In, you might decide to plan a potluck dinner in which everyone brings a dish for a special meal that creatively comes to 500 calories a person—including a predinner glass of wine and appetizers. As you experiment with your diet in a culinary way, you'll find recipes for drinks, appetizers, and delicious meals you can make in Chapters 9 and 11.

Make getting together with your girlfriends and having fun a habit, just like eating more fruits and vegetables! Put it on your meeting agenda: *What did you do last week to have fun?* Maybe you invited your BFF on a Sunday hike, involved the gals in the neighborhood in a before-the-day-starts jog, recruited the women at the dog park to do a weekly pooch walk or hit the farmers' market with your neighbor to scour for some interesting veggies. You'll score much-needed face time and cross something off your list.

Getting together for a weekly confab to keep each other on track and motivated is really only a small part of what your Girlfriends Diet Club can be. Girls' Nights Out can be great fun and a perfect way to free yourself from stress, but get-togethers don't always have to be about hanging at the bar or hitting the dance floor. So, what to do? Let your own interests and creativity be your guide. Here are just a few ideas that don't involve a bottle of wine:

* As a group, take up a charitable cause and spend evenings together working on a fund-raiser

* Does your driveway house a rarely used basketball hoop? Work in a little exercise and discuss the week while shooting baskets with your girlfriends.

* Turn one of your meetings into a potluck dinner and recipe exchange where you all bring a sampling of a new Mediterranean-style dish

* Get tickets to a play and spend time afterwards in lively discussion over a cocktail

* Have your group join in on a spin class—and have your meeting in the health club before or afterward

* Get a mani and a pedi together

* Plan a Sunday-afternoon scavenger hunt in which you follow the clues on foot and on bicycle

* Turn your diet club into a book club, too

"My girlfriends and I organize game nights. We play games like Bananagrams, Scrabble or Celebrity. We also have BBQ parties with our guys, where we get together and play Frisnoc, a Frisbee game we learned in college, but we created our own rules. It's a staple of almost every party we throw."

—*Ashley Schwartau, Nashville, TN*

Girls' Night Out

If you've canceled your umpteenth Girls Night Out and are feeling disconnected from your crew, add hangout time to your daily docket. You *can* take your diet out on the town. Weight-loss specialists warn that food has no place in a reward system for reaching weight-loss milestones—expert advice you should heed. If your diet club wants to reward individual achievements—two sizes lost, a 10K finish—don't turn it into a happy-hour celebration or gift card to P.F. Chang's. A belt to show off a thinner waist or a gift card for a few yoga sessions is a better idea.

But let's get real. Having dinner out is also fun. So here's how to do it without sabotaging your good food intentions. Start by getting in the habit of checking out restaurant websites before dining out. Even if a restaurant doesn't divulge nutrition information online, you can check out the menu and decide what you want before you head out. This way, you'll avoid making an impulse decision when you're there and feeling hungry. Key go-for-it menu hints: grilled, steamed, baked and broiled. Not-so-safe: crispy, creamy and cheesy. Ideal go-to staples are broth-based soups, salads and grilled chicken or fish with veggies.

The Skinny on the American Steak House

Steak houses, with their penchant for over-the-top portions— 40-ounce steaks, two-pound baked potatoes—seem more like a guy kind of place, but they are actually a safe haven for your diet. The reason? The à la carte selections allow you to order around the menu. A salad, a jumbo shrimp cocktail and a side of spinach, and you're set! You're out of there for around 500 calories or less, cocktail or wine included.

Shrimp cocktail is the ultimate guilt-free appetizer. Six jumbo shrimp come in at a mere 84 calories, and you can figure ¼ cup of cocktail sauce is 100 calories. Better yet, go for a half-dozen raw oysters. A medium oyster is only *10 calories*—and it's such a decadent treat. A cup of steamed spinach—OK, you'll be served maybe four cups—is only 42 calories as long as you skip the "creamed" choice. As for the salad, get the dressing—nothing creamy—on the side. A dressed salad can be a diet disaster.

If you simply can't go without an entrée, look for a petite filet mignon. Not a steak fan? Go for scallops (no cream sauce), a sure-bet low-calorie choice at only 156 calories for a *half pound* before add-ins, or a grilled piece of fish. Knock back on the large portions by sharing two or three entrées for the table. The waiter may frown, but, hey, it's your party!

Italian—Beware the Carbs

As restaurant food goes, pasta is cheap, so it costs the restaurateur only a few pennies per person to be extra generous filling your bowl. The result: too many carbs per serving! So if you decide to order pasta as your main dish, make sure you take home a doggie bag. For toppers, always choose a tomato-based option and skip anything named alfredo, vodka or anything with even a hint that there could be cream in it. One girlfriend weighed her doggie bag when she got home from a trendy trattoria, and it was a little over a pound. That's enough for four people!

Better yet, get the pasta as a side to a grilled chicken or fish dish. Remember, pasta is 220 calories a cup, so look at your plate and *visualize*. Measure out a cup at home and plop it on the plate so you get an idea. If you don't see whole wheat or a whole-grain pasta on the menu, ask for it. Even if the restaurant doesn't have it on the menu, many keep alternatives in the kitchen for special requests.

Another eater-beware area of caution is the bread basket. The big trend these days at Italian-style restaurants is to plop a basket of rolls and a little bowl of EVOO (extra-virgin olive oil) in front of you the moment you sit down. A nice healthy gesture, but one study that measured fat consumption found that diners eat less bread but too much fat when EVOO is on the table. So be careful not to soak up too much olive oil. Short-circuit the temptation to fall in the same boat by immediately ordering an app while you're looking at the

GF WANTS TO KNOW

I always try to watch my diet, but I have gained a few pounds, I think from my girls' nights out when, for some reason, my guard goes down and I go overboard. Got any advice?

—Getting Pudgy in Destin, FL

Dear GF,

Boy, girlfriend, do we ever know just what you mean! Those cocktails and apps will get you every time. In fact, because the whole point is to have a good time, many GFs tell us they save up during the day for the big night to come. Bad thinking—that strategy will only backfire.

Though it seems counterintuitive, the first thing you should do is eat a light, healthy snack *before* going out. It will keep you from inhaling high-calorie happy-hour nibbles like tortilla chips and nuts, or from munching on bread while you're looking over the menu. You'll also be in the mind-set of, *Hey, I feel good about my healthy pre-party snack, so why ruin it!*

If all your skinny girlfriends are ordering appetizers, make yours a salad, so when plates get passed around, you won't be tempted for more than just a nibble.

As for alcohol, stick with wine, light beer or single shots mixed with club soda. Even safer: A white-wine spritzer, which is wine mixed with a little clubby. (We offer plenty of low-cal ideas starting on page 206.)

And don't forget to mix some calorie-burning, body-moving activity into girls' night out, such as dancing or going from place to place on foot.

menu—either minestrone (vegetable-based clear soup that's about 80 calories) or a side salad with a non-creamy dressing on the side.

Japanese—A Low-Calorie Roll

Sushi is fun to do with a crowd and it's a popular Girlfriends choice because it's an opportunity to, shall we say, pig out while keeping the lid on calories—well, hopefully. Let's do some mental math. Keep calories low by starting with superlight and nutritious miso soup (about 80 calories a cup) or seaweed salad (about 100 calories). Share some really healthy and trendy edamame, but don't go overboard. Soybeans may be zero fat and good for you, but every half cup is 100 calories.

A sushi entrée can weigh in at a measly 200 calories or go over the top at 1,000, depending on what you order. What you should be cautious about is the rice, which gives you both calories—as much as is found in three slices of bread—and refined carbs. Add rice to your entrée, and you can almost double the calories.

Ever watch those guys prepare a sushi roll? A fascinating art, but they can pack a cup of rice in and around that seaweed. That's 200 calories *before* you add the fish, veggies and sauce. Ask for brown rice—it's becoming more popular—for a nutritional boost. If you're going to order sushi rolls, plan to share. Salmon, tuna, and yellowtail are all staples of the sushi bar and are among the leanest protein you can eat. Keep the calories down by ordering a vegetable roll or two in your group selection.

Avoid "Americanized" versions of sushi—such as a surf-and-turf roll, potato roll or the ones named after the sushi chef—which tend to have more fat and calories. As a rule of thumb, the more words that are used to describe the roll, the more fattening it is. Cream cheese and mayo jack up the calorie count, as do spicy rolls and salmon skins. Stay away from menu items billed as tempura, spider, dynamite or crunch—code for deep-fried. Diet-smart shrimp can ratchet up to 500 calories when they're part of a shrimp tempura roll.

Sushi without rice is called sashimi, and ordering it will give you about an ounce of protein and 35 calories per piece. Deliciously not bad!

"I make sure to order first in a restaurant, so I won't be tempted by what the others are having."

—*Kimberly Benhase Farrell,*
facebook.com/Goodhousekeeping

Chinese—Full Steam Ahead

Dining Chinese-style can be a deliciously lean experience as long as you know how to recognize the pitfalls while navigating the menu. Steamed anything—fish, vegetables, rice, noodles—will keep you right on course, but the same thing fried or "crispy" is a calorie land mine. That means skipping the egg roll at about 325 calories. A better idea when it comes to appetizers is ordering soup with 100 calories or less—egg drop, hot and sour, or wonton. Wontons and steamed dumplings are just 25 calories a pop.

Chinese entrées are meant for sharing, so have fun ordering a variety. Portions tend to be large, so order fewer entrées than you have diners—a must if you're going to be grazing on appetizers. Good, lower-calorie choices include steamed, broiled or roasted chicken, beef, pork or shrimp. Chow mein, chop suey, and moo goo gai pan are all safe choices because they also have lots of steamed veggies. Steer clear of anything described as crispy, coated, marinated, twice-cooked or battered. We're talking fat city. If you really want to be calorie frugal, ask for the sauce on the side.

There's one "crunchy" that you can take without guilt: the fortune cookie. They're only about 25 calories each—and who can resist finding out what their future may hold.

Mexican—Si, Si, Amiga

Nachos, burritos, chimichangas. So high in fat! Many people just love having Mexican, and if it is a to-die-for cuisine treat for your group, here's how to make it work for you.

Super-healthy guacamole and not-so-healthy chips are a common munchie for cruising the menu, but with so many calories and fat on the menu, it's best to let the guac go in favor of low-cal salsa. Just count out four or five chips each, and send the rest back to the kitchen.

Salads are fair game in most places, but not necessarily in a cantina. Really, where else do you go where you're supposed to eat the actual salad bowl! But it's not just the greasy shell. Most taco salads are smothered in fatty toppings that can pile upwards of 1,000 calories. Give it the red light.

Go green, instead, with posole, a yummy Latin broth-based soup featuring hominy, a fiber-filled member of the corn family. It usually contains veggies, some pork and chili peppers and is one of the lighter selections on the menu at about 175 calories. Couple it with seviche, which is fresh fish or shrimp marinated with diced vegetables and plenty of lime juice to "cook" the fish, for another 175 calories or so.

Tacos can be a safe bet as long as the shell is *soft*—not fried—and you have chicken or fish. Pile on the salsa, but skip the cheese, sour cream and guacamole, and you're looking at about 200 calories each. Add some jalapeños to amp up the heat. Spicy foods help fill you up and they may even boost your metabolism. (For more on this, see page 115.)

A tostada is a crispy corn taco wrapped around beans, meat, cheese and salsa. Ordinarily, this kind of pileup could lead to a heap of trouble, but it can't really hold too much, so you can probably keep the lid at around 300 calories.

And the final Mexican restaurant tip: Go for corn tortillas over flour. They have about half the calories and twice the fiber, making them a better option in every instance. If you're making Mexican at home, you can use taco-size whole wheat or corn tortillas.

The Girl-Friendly Bar

It's always 5 o'clock somewhere, and if it's the bar where you and your girlfriends are, you want to make sure you don't end up drinking all the calories you have left for the day. Diet wisdom tells us to spend all of our daily calories on food and to only quaff beverages with zero calories. Great advice when it comes to quenching your thirst or washing down your lunch, but impossible when you're out for a night on the town.

Keep in mind that drinking can pack on the pounds and railroad even the best-laid dieting strategy. For many women, boozing makes them hungry. It also loosens inhibitions, so your plan to get the salad and a light entrée may fall by the wayside. However, Girlfriends can still enjoy a drink (or occasionally two) without tipping the scale by planning and budgeting their drinking calories.

It's really easy—just a little arithmetic. When you know you're doing a Girls' Night Out or date night, plan ahead. Decide what you're going to drink and figure out the calories. Then, simply trim back the same amount of calories through food during the day. That can't be too hard when you choose your booze wisely and limit yourself to one. Smart girl choices:

 * White wine spritzer (5 oz.)—60 calories

 * Champagne (4 oz.)—90 calories

 * Wine (5 oz.)—120 calories

* Tequila on the rocks with a splash of seltzer and a
  squeeze of lime (1.5 oz.)—120 calories

* Vodka and club soda with a splash of cranberry juice
  (5 oz.)—130 calories

These days designer cocktails are all the rage, but they probably
won't do your calorie budget any favors. If the ingredients of
Marshall's Manhattan Martini aren't described on the menu, ask
the barkeep what's in it, and act accordingly. The rule of thumb:
The simpler, the better. Here's a sample of smart and not-so-smart
offerings you're liable to see on a menu:

✓ SMART: POMEGRANATE MARTINI

A 4-oz. serving made with flavored vodka and pure pomegranate
juice (about half of each) has about 185 calories. The juice packs a
ton of flavor, plus a punch of antioxidants.

✗ NOT SO SMART: CHOCOLATE MARTINI

Figure in the sugary chocolate syrup and some heavy cream to
make it smooth and—*yikes!*—you're downing anywhere from 300
to 500 calories. Who wants to drink dessert anyway.

✓ SMART: RED WINE

A glass of red wine, about 120 calories for five ounces, is meant
for sipping, so it can last you all the way through dinner.

✓✓ EVEN SMARTER: SANGRIA

The combination of wine, fruit and club soda can bring the wine
calorie count down to 80 calories.

✓ SMART: BLOODY MARY

A tall glass with nutritious tomato juice, yummy spices, a jigger of

vodka and a zap of metabolism-boosting heat is just 125 calories—
and that's counting the celery stick!

✗✗ JUST SAY NO: LONG ISLAND ICED TEA

The boozy concoction of vodka, gin, rum, tequila and triple sec,
topped off with a little O.J. is more than a meal at about 800 calories, if you—*hiccup*—make it to the bottom of the glass.

Girls Go Wild

When Nancy Wilson and Betty Tack wanted to celebrate 30 years of
friendship and their recent weight loss, they headed for a yoga and
health retreat in Massachusetts' Berkshire Mountains to get out of
their comfort zone and do some mental retooling.

The first afternoon they signed up for a class called the Journey
Dance, which was not so much physically challenging as it was mentally. The instructor guided them through dance sequences in which
they were asked to imagine themselves as trees, then as cats, and at
the pinnacle of silliness, they were engaging in a brief "bumper butt"
dance with other people whom they'd never met.

"We felt like we were violating some unwritten law against grown
women engaging in loony behavior, and had to work hard not to
bolt out of the room," recalls Wilson. "But then something shifted,
and by the end of the 'journey,' we were enjoying ourselves." They
lost track of time; they shed their intimidation; they were having fun.

We can all use an escape once in a while that offers us a new
adventure and some life-assuring self-confidence. When you are
planning a Girlfriends Weekend be sure to include *plenty* of group
activities—hiking, walking, biking, yoga on the beach—in addition
to just sitting around and enjoying the scenery and just talking. And
when you take your diet on vacation, make it something that will

Girl-Friendliest Brews

Our image through male eyes may have us sipping white wine or some pink frozen drink with an umbrella floater, but recent polls show that 27% of us are beer lovers. Yet, beer guts are so unbecoming! We recruited a small band of beer-drinking GFs for an impromptu party to find the tastiest brews with the lowest calories per bottle. These five floated to the top:

Yuengling Light Lager. *99 calories, 8.8 grams of carbs.* Our brewsters were won over by its spiciness and found it "flavorful and full-bodied." Definitely the go-to for a Girls' Night Out or Girls' Night In party.

Amstel Light. *95 calories, 5 grams of carbs.* You can't beat the classics! Our GFs loved the "golden color" and "slight sweetness" of this "smooth" lager. It could even pass for full-metal beer. Said one sipper: "Only 95 calories? No way!"

MGD 64. *64 calories, 2.4 grams of carbs.* That's code for Miller Genuine Draft tuned down. GFs were floored by how much rich, malty favor is packed into each bottle. It was "not bitter or watery" like others that didn't make the final five.

Michelob Ultra Pomegranate Raspberry. *95 calories, 5.5 grams of carbs.* The hands-down favorite among Michelob's three fruity beers and the perfect low-cal alternative for fans of Belgian framboise and other berry-infused brews.

Select 55. *55 calories, 1.9 grams of carbs.* As low as you can go and still call it beer! The lighest beer on the shelves is surprisingly crisp and refreshing with a nice flavor. It's a slam-dunk for calorie counters.

supercharge your willpower, reinforce your commitment to a healthy lifestyle and bond your relationships with a lifetime of memories. The ultimate reward: Returning home relaxed and enriched, and to a scale that's actually moved down.

For you and your girlfriends, it might just be a hike in the woods or a trip to the spa or the beach. Do whatever floats your boat, but set out to make it something active and engaging. We may not all have the luxury or even the time for what we might consider the ultimate escape, but knowing it exists and dreaming about it can still

AMAZING! MAKEOVER

Sarah Elizabeth Richards
"What I Miss About Being Fat."

I STOOD AT THE BAR, awkwardly clutching my margarita. My two girlfriends were chatting up a mechanical engineer and his cousin. Feeling left out, I tried to make eye contact with a cute guy by the door. He ignored me.

This was not how I imagined my big new-body debut. I was newly single after a breakup with a longtime boyfriend, and my friends had persuaded me to join them at the kitschy bar where, they promised, I would meet fun, desirable men.

I had recently lost 40 pounds—mostly by upping my intake of vegetables and whole grains and cutting out sugar, pasta and white bread—and had taken my friends' advice to wear clothes that showed off my body—a carefully selected neon-pink chiffon top, a short black skirt and high heels. Telling me I looked hot, my friends assured me I'd get hit on.

The air-conditioning was cranked up, and I felt the cold air on every inch of exposed skin—my bare arms, legs, cleavage and collarbone, which finally had reappeared after years of being encased in fat. But instead of feeling sexy, I felt naked.

"I'm really tired," I told my friends. "I'm going to go."

Back home, I opened my closet and found my old fat clothes: the cavernous yoga pants and faded sweatshirt with the holes near the armpits. I buried my face in them and took in the mix of lingering perfume and detergent. I put them on, my anxiety subsiding. I felt like me again.

Sometimes I missed my fat. People always talk about the benefits of weight loss, but there's little discussion about the sheer shock of it. When you first decide to diet, you imagine only the upsides: new body, better health. No one warns you how rattled you'll feel. Physically, I was perpetually cold and dogged by a dull ache underneath my rib cage— the sensation I experienced whenever I felt vulnerable. Emotionally, I felt ill-equipped to handle all of the changes, and I could no longer turn to the comfort foods that soothed me.

Then there was the disappointment. In my thin fantasies, I was more confident and better dressed. I had more friends and dates. I pushed myself professionally. Sometimes I slow danced at garden parties in sexy sheaths while my imaginary boyfriend nuzzled my neck. When I was fat, these fantasies stayed safely in the realm of "someday."

And the smaller version wasn't necessarily a better one—at least not at first. I loved my newly visible collarbone and the emerging curve on my lower back, but I never imagined that I would stand naked in front of the mirror, grabbing rolls of loose skin from under my arms and inner thighs. Or that I would see my breasts become floppy and flat or my butt even more dimpled. I felt like a stranger in my own body.

There was also the day-to-day stuff. Diet experts don't tell you how left out you feel when you're unable to share the platter of penne alla vodka or pitchers of beer with friends. Or how nearly every interaction includes a reference to your new size. My friends were always encouraging me with flattering comments as the weight was coming off. At first I enjoyed hearing, "Look at you, Miss Skinny!" But sometimes I didn't want the attention; I just wanted the comfort of the group.

I didn't actually want my fat back; I had worked hard to lose it. For most of my adult life, I carried an extra five to 20 pounds, but during graduate school I topped out at 180 on my 5'6" frame by ordering takeout lasagna and pad Thai to get through the mountains of work. I wore

"Seeing my friends and how comfortable they were in these clothes taught me that I didn't need to be perfect to wear them, either."

loose clothing and had little idea how much I had gained until I stepped on a doctor's scale.

Today, I'm 140 pounds, a weight I've maintained for about four years. It took me nearly seven years to get there. It wasn't because I regained the weight. I just couldn't bear to drop it any faster than five to seven pounds at a time. The slow weight loss, it turns out, was actually good for my body. It also gave my initially loose skin time to catch up. Yoga and kickboxing did the rest. But the reason for my slow-poke pace was that I needed months to get used to each new size—and identity. As soon as my clothes were too big, the loss would stall, which I'd blame on my body's natural plateau. Now, I believe I ate just enough to keep my weight the same because I'd reached my comfort level.

The last 15 pounds took almost three years. I would lose a couple here and there, but I was never too serious, reluctant to give up my status as an "almost thin" person. At 155 pounds, I could safely peer into a world in which my friends wore halter tops and bikinis, while I was getting used to loose tank tops. I was still trying to tolerate that naked feeling. They didn't always have the perfect body for what they were wearing, but they still looked good and they felt confident in what they were wearing. I just wasn't feeling the same way about me in the same kinds of clothes. Seeing my friends and how comfortable they were in these clothes taught me that I didn't need to be perfect to wear them, either.

I wish I could say I learned to feel good through some organic process of loving myself—by celebrating my strengths, accepting my flaws. Rather, I forced myself to feel good incrementally, like easing myself into a cold pool. Over the next few years, I invented little assignments for myself. I bought form-fitting tank tops for the gym. At first, I wore them only inside the dark spinning studio. Then, for the next couple of months, I wore them inside the brightly lit workout rooms but stood in the back. Eventually, I

"I bought form-fitting tank tops for the gym. . . Eventually I watched myself do bicep curls in front of the mirror."

watched myself do bicep curls in full view of the mirrors. On a vacation in South Beach, I even experimented with a bikini. Reclining on a lounge chair, I lifted my white linen cover-up to expose my belly to the sun. By the end of the trip, I'd made myself take it off and walk to the pool.

One of the mistakes I made at first was trying to put my social life on hold while I was losing weight. That doesn't work. You can't say *no* to your friends all the time in the hope that you'll be able to say *yes* when you get to be the image you have in your head. That's not workable. Just make a decision to eat healthfully and go with it. You can go out and have fun, just learn to budget your calories.

I still wrestle with that naked feeling, but it doesn't overwhelm me and make me run home from bars and my GFs anymore. On the rare occasions that it gets unbearable, I wrap myself in a big terrycloth robe until it passes. And it always does. Then I put on my new fitted yoga pants, which hug my beautiful curves.

be part of the fun. Here are some things Girlfriends have done and places they have gone, and how they sized up the experience. Pick a few and put them on your dream list.

"Fun for me is always somewhat removed from my normal reality. I like running through the mountains with a camera, stopping to take photographs along the way, or doing karaoke. The more active the experience, the more playful I feel—and it enables me to get out of my own way."

—*Hyla Molander, Tiburon, CA*

Spas and Wellness Escapes

Ahhhhh! Just the thought of it feels so relaxing. During the past few decades, the number and assortment of spas—and the things to do at them—have expanded by leaps and bounds. If you're looking for a spa experience, chances are you won't have to travel too far from home. Just be sure to do your homework first.

To make it diet-friendly, you'll want your spa escape to be more than massages, facials and mud baths. Pick a place that will get you plenty of movement, too. Your reward at the end of each day—at least at most places—will be chef-prepared gourmet-style dinners that are super-healthy.

The spa experience is extremely diverse so think of what you and your girlfriends enjoy and the challenges you might what to meet. For example, you get an experiential cowboy-country vacation combined with luxe-yet-rugged pampering at Travaasa in Austin, TX (travaasa.com/austin), where you can ease in with yoga and a Texas two-step lesson, venture into climbing along the Prickly Pear Challenge Course and—not to be missed—try the mechanical-bull workout. It's a Zen-like preserve for the soul.

If riding is in your blood, head to the Salamander Resort & Spa in Middleburg, VA (salamanderresort.com). Jackie O. and Liz Taylor used to ride in style at this 340-acre resort, which now boasts balance and strength stations set up on the edge of the nature preserve and an over-the-top 23,000-square-foot spa that has terraces adorned with massage spaces, plus tree-house treatment rooms.

If you're really taking your diet seriously and love to cook, you might want to head for a three-day escape to the Ramekins Culinary School and Inn in Sonoma, CA (ramekins.com), where you will raise a glass (or two) to your health. In addition to the traditional spa experience, you'll tour a sustainable farm, learn winemaking and enjoy breathtaking views. You'll also go home with a new repertoire of healthy recipes that will truly make you the hostess with the mostest.

Rest and Recreation Retreats

OK, the rest comes after the recreation, but these retreats put the emphasis on treats, as in luxury accommodations and everything-at-your-fingertips amenities, from top-of-the-line equipment to top-notch guides. For example, girlfriends reported back that the bunk beds never looked so plush as they did at Basecamp Hotel South Lake Tahoe in Lake Tahoe, CA (basecamphotels.com), a boutique hotel for those with an explorer's spirit. You'll spend your days skiing, snowboarding, snowshoeing and sledding along the trails, mountains and lakes of the Lake Tahoe Basin, and your nights in the hotel's cozy communal space, where fellow explorers share stories, two fire pits with s'mores kits and an in-house Instagram feed to post the day's best images.

If the desert's more to your liking, you might want to head to the Four Seasons Resort Rancho Encantado in Santa Fe, NM (encantadoresort.com), where you can rediscover your inner artist under the grand skies and infinite stars of this high-mountain 57-acre wellness resort. Check out the Outdoor & Cultural Pursuits program, where expert guides take you on exclusive adventures tailored to your group's fitness level. The truly adventurous might want to try the geocoaching package, a treasure hunt that works your GPS to the hilt and takes you through landmarks in downtown Santa Fe or the Sangre de Cristo Mountains. Your reward will be trimmer thighs and slimmer hips, even on five-star-quality food.

If doing your own thing at your own pace is more your thing, you might want to head for a place like the Hotel Vermont in Burlington, VT (hotelvt.com), where you can experience rugged New England charm with a lot of local flavor. The menu showcases what's flourishing right outside, and rooms are fashioned from Vermont oak and marble. Hike the Green Mountains, take sailing lessons on Lake

Champlain, do morning yoga, go on a bike ride along country roads and enjoy a before-bedtime hot stone message.

If you love the great outdoors, head for a place like The Resort at

Paws Up in Greenough, MT (pawsup.com), a 37,000-acre working ranch (yes, 37,000) with "glamping" accommodations and gorgeous views of Big Sky Country. Ah, wilderness! It's real cowgirl culture, where you'll saddle up for a cattle drive, then wind down at the tented Spa Town, which offers yoga and quirkily named massages (Cowboy Classic, Sacagawea's Dream). Best of all, you'll sleep under the stars—next to a roaring, butler-prepped fire.

Big Adventure Destinations

For the ultimate girlfriends' challenge, sign up for an *Amazing Race*–style competition. If you want to feel the pounds melt off, this is the way. If you have the time and the money and want a real escape, try something like Hawaiian Seascapes (adventuresmithexplorations .com), a seven-day 36-person yachting expedition to the remote, accessible-by-sea-only coves and jungles of Maui, Molokai, Lanai,

Molokini and the Big Island of Hawaii. You will be able to swim, snorkel, scuba, paddle and whale-watch in these unusually spectacular places. Girlfriends report once-in-a-lifetime experiences like net fishing with the natives—and having the chef prepare your catch for dinner—helping to restore an ancient taro field and riding a mule down a steep hill to Father Damien's legendary sanctuary. Authentic luaus and massages are included in the cost.

A little closer to home (and reality) for most of us is the even more challenging New Balance Reach the Beach Relay Race: Mountain Creek to Island Beach, NJ (rtbrelay.com), and other locations. It's the ultimate team relay running challenge: 200 miles over the course of 24 hours with the help of 11 friends. The scenery features darling historic towns, majestic state parks and—for a splashy finale—the shores of Island Beach. At the finish line, there's massage, music, food and an invigorated sense of camaraderie. Check online for dates.

There are even ways you can combine adventure with learning something new. An experience one girls' group recommends is learning photography with Far and Away Adventures' Photography Safari on the Middle Fork of the Salmon River, ID (theamericansafari. com). It combines small-group workshops with a luxury rafting adventure through stunning landscapes that earned the region a spot in *1,000 Places to See Before You Die*. The level of luxury peaks with chef-prepared organic dinners, riverside massages, luxe tents, solar-heated showers—and the assurance that for once you'll go home with photos that do your trip justice.

GF Action Plan

The Girlfriends Diet is a new way of life that includes taking time for yourself and remembering (without guilt) to put yourself before others at least once in a while. It also means not putting life "on hold" when we're on "a diet." So, on a frequent basis—try to shoot for at least once a week—give yourself permission to have fun:

ADD SOMETHING FUN FOR *YOU* TO YOUR TO-DO LIST. Remember this is something for you—not the kids, spouse or boss!

TAKE YOUR DIET OUT ON THE TOWN with your girlfriends so you can all learn together how to have fun and stay within the parameters of your diet. Stay active together.

PLAN A SPECIAL GETAWAY. Use it to celebrate a special milestone you or your diet club has achieved on The Girlfriends Diet.

* Order a copy of *The Girlfriends Diet* for your friend at goodhousekeeping.com/girlfriends.
* Share your success stories and get more dieting tips on our Facebook page at facebook.com/girlfriendsdiet.

PART 2

The Girlfriends Meal Plan & Recipes

chapter 8 The Meal Plan

HERE IS A FOUR-WEEK SAMPLE of what you can eat following the parameters of The Girlfriends Diet Mediterranean-style plan, based on having 1,400 to 1,600 calories a day. The plan gives you three meals adding up to 1,300 calories plus 100 to 300 calories for snacks and/or a glass of wine. This is the range most women will fall into when they cut back 500 to 1,000 calories a day in order to lose one or two pounds a week. If your burn rate allows you to consume more calories, there are 100- and 200-calorie options for additional snacks or you can include another side dish with the appropriate calorie count to supplement the basic meal plan. Just remember not to exceed your total daily calorie consumption represented by your personal RMR that you figured out from the formulas in Chapter 2, minus the number of calories you are cutting back to achieve your weight loss goal.

These menu plans show you what a typical week can look like when you're eating approximately 50% carbohydrates; 30% fat, with only 10% from saturated fat; and 20% protein for the day. We believe it's the ideal breakdown of nutrients that helps promote weight loss in women. Use the recipes in the following chapters as your guide as you learn adapt to this style of eating.

Remember, as long as you fill half your plate with veggies and fruit, one-quarter with whole grains and the rest with some protein—a little meat and the rest plant-based (such as beans)—at each of your main meals, you'll be on track. And you don't have to worry about fat because the meal plan was developed to come in at under 30% fat and 10% saturated fat.

The meal plan that starts on the next page is flexible. Each week's meals have been balanced and provide the vitamins and nutrients you need while avoiding consecutive days that feature overlapping ingredients or flavors. Feel free to substitute any breakfast for any other breakfast. And since all lunches and dinners are about 500 calories, you can swap these meals as well. Make sure to keep track of the calories for everything you are eating and drinking and enjoy the wonderful meals that come from eating the Mediterranean-style foods featured in The Girlfriends Diet.

Week 1 ||||||||||||||||||||||||||||||||||||||||||||||||||||||||||||||||||||||||||||||||||||||||||||||||

DAY	BREAKFAST	LUNCH	DINNER
1	Figgy Waffle page 228	Souper Soup **Side:** Pear page 240	Greek Chicken **Side:** Roasted Asparagus & Whole Wheat Orzo page 250
2	Kale Smoothie page 229	Burger Day **Side:** Hummus & Veggie Dippers page 236	Halibut with Tomato, Olive & Pine Nut Relish **Side:** Steamed Spinach & Quinoa page 255
3	Baklava Yogurt page 227	Greek Grain Salad page 239	Feta Turkey Burgers with Yogurt Mint Sauce **Side:** Mushroom Soup & Sweet Potato Fries page 249
4	Spicy Egg Sandwich page 230	Chicken, Spinach & Strawberry Salad **Side:** Triscuits page 237	Vegetable Lasagna Toss **Side:** Salad page 274
5	Grainy Breakfast Bowl page 228	Nut Butter Sandwich **Side:** Strawberries with Greek Yogurt Dip page 240	Italian Steak Kabobs **Dessert:** Fire-Roasted Nectarines with Berry Salsa page 257
6	Grab & Go page 228	California Chicken Sandwich **Side:** SunChips **Dessert:** Apple page 237	Sticky Glazed Salmon **Side:** Steamed Baby Carrots & Quinoa with Almonds page 269
7	Morning Glory Muffin **Side:** Yogurt and Strawberries page 234	Asian Tuna Salad **Side:** Ak-Mak Crackers page 236	Black Bean Soup **Side:** Multigrain Tortilla Chips page 242

Week 2 ||||||||||||||||||||||||||||||||||||||||||||||||||||||||||||||||||

DAY	BREAKFAST	LUNCH	DINNER
1	Tropical Oatmeal & Fruit Salad page 230	Panera Bread Takeout **Dessert:** Apple page 240	Chicken Salad with Orzo & Feta **Dessert:** Grapes page 247
2	Morning Glory Muffin **Side:** Yogurt and Strawberries page 234	Nachos page 239	Grilled Portabello Burger with Pesto Mayo **Dessert:** Watermelon page 253
3	Sweet Potato Hash page 230	Mediterranean Wrap **Side:** Grapes page 239	Penne with Escarole, White Beans & Toasted Bread Crumbs page 262
4	Broiled Grapefruit page 228	Tuna Bean Salad **Side:** Ak-Mak Crackers page 241	Lemon Oregano Roasted Chicken **Side:** Roasted Sweet Potatoes page 259
5	Cereal Bowl page 228	Cheese Plate page 237	Spicy Tuna Roll Salad page 268
6	Artichoke Frittata page 231	Burger Day **Side:** Hummus & Veggie Dippers page 236	Classic Minestrone **Side:** Whole Wheat Dinner Roll page 268
7	Overnight Balsamic Berry Salad page 229	Chicken Sandwich **Side:** Baby Carrots & Sweet Potato Chips **Dessert:** Orange page 237	Hoisin-Glazed Salmon with Quinoa page 256

Week 3

DAY	BREAKFAST	LUNCH	DINNER
1	Whole-Grain Pancakes page 235	Spinach Salad Pita page 240	Lamb Lollichops with Wine Sauce **Side:** Spinach Sauté **Dessert:** Clementine page 258
2	Morning Muesli page 229	Greek Salad **Side:** Whole Wheat Pita page 238	Pasta with Goat Cheese & Walnuts **Side:** Roasted Broccoli page 261
3	Breakfast Pizza page 227	Butternut Squash Soup **Dessert:** Pear & Graham Cracker page 236	Chicken & Mushrooms with Brown Rice **Dessert:** Buttermilk Panna Cotta with Blackberry Sauce page 245
4	Pumpkin Whoopie Pie page 229	Mediterranean Grilled Cheese **Dessert:** Kiwi page 239	Tuna Tomato Linguini page 270
5	Kale Smoothie page 229	Black Bean & Corn Salad **Side:** Multigrain Tortilla Chips page 236	Chicken with Arugula Pesto Spaghetti page 246
6	Cheddar & Chicken Omelet page 233	Asian Tuna Salad **Side:** Ak-Mak Crackers page 236	Moroccan Style Chickpea & Sweet Potato Stew **Dessert:** Brandy-Poached Winter Fruit with Cinnamon & Star Anise page 260
7	Apple Cinnamon Oatmeal page 227	Grapefruit & Avocado Salad **Side:** Whole Wheat Dinner Roll page 238	Greek-Style Stuffed Peppers **Side:** Roasted Beet & Olive Salad with Orange & Mint **Dessert:** Chocolate Pudding Cake page 251

Week 4 ||||||||||||||||||||||||||||||||||||||||||||||||||||||||||||||||||||||

DAY	BREAKFAST	LUNCH	DINNER
1	PB&J Waffle Sandwich page 229	Chicken Sandwich **Side:** Baby Carrots & Sweet Potato Chips **Dessert:** Orange page 237	Pizza Crust Panzanella **Dessert:** Melon with Prosciutto page 263
2	Sweet Potato Hash page 230	Chicken, Spinach & Strawberry Salad **Side:** Triscuits page 237	Tuscan Sun Salmon Salad **Side:** Focaccia page 273
3	Baklava Yogurt page 227	Nachos page 239	Quick Chicken Kebabs **Side:** Brown Rice with Red Peppers page 264
4	Broiled Grapefruit page 228	Easy Caesar Salad **Side:** Whole-Grain Roll **Dessert:** Cherries page 238	Red Cabbage Spaghetti with Golden Raisins **Dessert:** Grapes page 265
5	Cereal Bowl page 228	Mediterranean Wrap **Dessert:** Grapes page 239	Beef & Bulgur Falafel **Side:** Spinach Sauté page 241
6	Asparagus & Cheese Frittata page 232	Tuna Bean Salad **Side:** Ak-Mak Crackers page 241	Buttermilk Oven-Fried Chicken Tenders **Side:** Butternut Squash Fries **Dessert:** Apple Crisp page 244
7	Whole-Grain Pancakes page 235	DiGiorno **Side:** Salad page 238	Turkey Vegetable Soup **Side:** Open-Faced Cheese Toast with Avocado page 291

chapter 9 Recipes for Every Meal

TUSCAN SUN SALMON SALAD. Halibut with Tomato, Olive & Pine Nut Relish. Tropical Oatmeal & Fruit Salad. Just the sound of these Mediterranean-style dishes that are part and parcel of The Girlfriends Diet are enough to make you want to dig in!

The more than 150 recipes in this section—300-calorie breakfasts, 500-calorie lunches, 500-calorie dinners, appetizers, side dishes, snacks, desserts and even cocktails—were designed with busy women in mind. They are so easy to follow because all of the breakfasts, lunches and dinners are complete meals. The breakfasts and lunches are all designed as single servings unless otherwise noted, while the serving sizes for dinners indicate how many people the dish will serve. The recipes also spotlight the foods in The Girlfriends Diet Food Basket that will help you get more acquainted with the Mediterranean style of eating.

At the end of each recipe, you will find nutritional information so you'll be able to keep track of your calories and other nutrients. While sodium is not a focus of The Girlfriends Diet, it is something that a lot of women monitor, so we've included information about it as well. The meal plan allows for less than 2,400 milligrams of sodium, which is in keeping with recommendations for healthy people.

Breakfasts—about 300 calories

APPLE-CINNAMON OATMEAL:

Cook ½ c. old-fashioned oats with ½ c. fat-free milk, ½ c. water, a pinch of cinnamon and a pinch of salt. Add ½ apple, chopped, and 1 Tbsp. chopped walnuts to cooked oatmeal. PER SERVING | Calories 300 | Protein 12 g | Carbohydrate 47 g | Total fat 8 g | Sat fat 0.5 g | Fiber 7 g | Sodium 11 mg

BAKLAVA YOGURT

Top 1 c. plain nonfat Greek yogurt with 1 shredded wheat biscuit, crumbled, 1 Tbsp. pistachios, shelled, ½ c. strawberries, sliced, and 1½ tsp. honey. PER SERVING | Calories 320 | Protein 29 g | Carbohydrate 45 g | Total fat 4.5 g | Sat fat 0 g | Fiber 6 g | Sodium 90 mg

BREAKFAST PIZZA

Scramble one egg in nonstick olive oil spray. Split and toast a small (4-in.) whole wheat pita and top with egg divided among both halves. Sprinkle each half with 2 Tbsp. reduced-fat Cheddar cheese, broil until Cheddar melts. Serve with 1 c. melon cubes. PER SERVING Calories 270 | Protein 14 g | Carbohydrate 30 g | Total fat 11 g | Sat fat 4.5 g | Fiber 3 g Sodium 440 mg

BROILED GRAPEFRUIT

Sprinkle 1 tsp. brown sugar over ½ grapefruit and broil for 2 to 3 minutes, until sugar gets bubbly. Serve with 1 slice whole wheat bread, toasted and spread with 1 Tbsp. nut butter. Have with a chai tea latte made with 1 chai tea bag and ½ c. heated fat-free milk.

PER SERVING | Calories 290 | Protein 13 g | Carbohydrate 42 g | Total fat 9 g | Sat fat 2 g
Fiber 5 g | Sodium 270 mg

CEREAL BOWL

Have 1 c. Multi-Grain Cheerios with 1 c. fat-free milk, ½ c. strawberries, halved, and 1 Tbsp. roasted almonds, chopped.

PER SERVING | Calories 270 | Protein 13 g | Carbohydrate 45 g | Total fat 6 g | Sat fat 0.5 g
Fiber 5 g | Sodium 340 mg

FIGGY WAFFLE

Top a toasted, whole-grain waffle (such as Kashi or Van's) with ⅓ c. part-skim ricotta, 2 dried figs, chopped, 1 Tbsp. chopped walnuts and 1 tsp. honey. PER SERVING | Calories 300 | Protein 14 g
Carbohydrate 35 g | Total fat 15 g | Sat fat 4.5 g | Fiber 6 g | Sodium 220 mg

GRAB & GO

Have one 16-oz. skim-milk, unsweetened latte from your favorite coffee shop with 15 almonds and 20 grapes. PER SERVING | Calories 330
Protein 17 g | Carbohydrate 39 g | Total fat 11 g | Sat fat 1 g | Fiber 3 g | Sodium 210 mg

GRAINY BREAKFAST BOWL

To ⅔ c. cooked quinoa (either leftover and heated or cooked in the morning), add 1½ Tbsp. chopped walnuts, ½ pear, chopped, a pinch of cinnamon, and 1 tsp. honey. PER SERVING | Calories 290 | Protein 7 g
Carbohydrate 48 g | Total fat 10 g | Sat fat 0.5 g | Fiber 7 g | Sodium 10 mg

KALE SMOOTHIE

Blend 1 c. baby kale, 1 c. frozen mango chunks, ½ c. plain nonfat Greek yogurt, ½ c. fat-free milk and 1 tsp. honey. Serve with 5 dry-roasted almonds. PER SERVING | Calories 310 | Protein 20 g

Carbohydrate 52 g | Total fat 4 g | Sat fat 0 g | Fiber 6 g | Sodium 140 mg

MORNING MUESLI

Mix ⅓ c. old-fashioned oats with 1 apple, chopped, ½ c. fat-free milk and a pinch of cinnamon. Refrigerate overnight, and in the morning, top with 1 Tbsp. chopped walnuts. PER SERVING | Calories 290

Protein 10 g | Carbohydrate 51 g | Total fat 7 g | Sat fat 0.5 g | Fiber 8 g | Sodium 55 mg

OVERNIGHT BALSAMIC BERRY SALAD

Mix 1 c. strawberries, halved, with 1 Tbsp. balsamic vinegar and 1 tsp. sugar; refrigerate at least 4 hrs. or overnight. In the morning, serve atop ⅓ c. part-skim ricotta. Serve with 1 slice whole wheat toast spread with 1 tsp. all-fruit preserve. PER SERVING | Calories 280

Protein 14 g | Carbohydrate 39 g | Total fat 8 g | Sat fat 4.5 g | Fiber 5 g | Sodium 250 mg

PB&J WAFFLE SANDWICH

Mix 1 Tbsp. peanut butter and 1 tsp. strawberry fruit preserves into 2 Tbsp. nonfat Greek yogurt. Spread between 2 toasted whole-grain waffles (such as Kashi or Van's). PER SERVING | Calories 300

Protein 15 g | Carbohydrate 42 g | Total fat 11 g | Sat fat 1.5 g | Fiber 7 g | Sodium 410 mg

PUMPKIN WHOOPIE PIE

Mix ½ tsp. pumpkin pie spice and 1 tsp. maple syrup into ¼ c. plain nonfat Greek yogurt. Toast 2 whole-grain waffles (such as Kashi or Van's) and spread Greek yogurt mixture on one and ¼ c. canned pumpkin on the other. Sandwich together. Serve with ½ banana. PER SERVING | Calories 290 | Protein 15 g | Carbohydrate 58 g | Total fat 3.5 g

Sat fat 0 g | Fiber 10 g | Sodium 360 mg

SPICY EGG SANDWICH

Scramble 1 egg in a skillet coated with olive oil cooking spray. Stir in ½ c. baby spinach until wilted. Put egg mixture on a toasted, 100% whole wheat English muffin along with ¼ avocado, sliced, and 1 tsp. sriracha. Serve with ½ c. cantaloupe chunks. PER SERVING Calories 310 | Protein 14 g | Carbohydrate 37 g | Total fat 13 g | Sat fat 2.5 g | Fiber 8 g Sodium 510 mg

SWEET POTATO HASH

Cook ½ red pepper, diced, and ¼ onion, diced, in a skillet with 1 tsp. extra-virgin olive oil; when vegetables are softened, add 1 egg and egg white, whisked, and scramble. Serve eggs atop 1 serving Alexia frozen sweet potato fries, cooked according to package directions. PER SERVING | Calories 300 | Protein 12 g | Carbohydrate 31 g | Total fat 15 g Sat fat 2 g | Fiber 5 g | Sodium 270 mg

TROPICAL OATMEAL & FRUIT SALAD

Mix ½ c. cubed melon with ½ c. cubed mango, ½ tsp. fresh mint, chopped, and a squirt of lime juice. Serve with 1 c. cooked oatmeal (prepared with water), and top with 2 tsp. unsweetened shredded coconut and 1 Tbsp. chopped walnuts. PER SERVING | Calories 300 Protein 7 g | Carbohydrate 54 g | Total fat 9 g | Sat fat 3 g | Fiber 8 g | Sodium 180 mg

Artichoke Frittata

MAKES **4 SERVINGS**

1 lb. sm. red potatoes, cut into quarters

1 Tbsp. plus 1 tsp. olive oil

⅜ tsp. salt

⅜ tsp. pepper

2 green onions, sliced

1 orange bell pepper (8 oz.), chopped

1 pt. grape tomatoes

1 can (13 to 14 oz.) artichoke hearts, rinsed and chopped

4 lg. eggs plus 4 lg. egg whites

½ c. crumbled feta cheese

1. Arrange oven rack 6 in. from broiler heat source. Preheat broiler.

2. To medium microwave-safe bowl, add potatoes and ¼ c. water; cover with vented plastic wrap. Microwave on High 8 min. or until tender. Drain. On baking sheet, toss potatoes with 1 tsp. oil and ⅛ tsp. each salt and pepper. Broil 6 min. or until browned.

3. Meanwhile, in nonstick 10-in. skillet, heat 1 Tbsp. oil on medium 1 min. Add green onions and orange pepper; cook 5 min. or until golden, stirring occasionally. Add tomatoes and artichoke hearts; cook 2 to 5 min. or until tomatoes start to burst, stirring occasionally.

4. While vegetables cook, in medium bowl, beat eggs and egg whites with ¼ tsp. each salt and pepper and half of feta. Pour over vegetables and tilt skillet to distribute. Top with remaining feta. Cover; cook 5 to 6 min. or until set. Serve with potatoes.

PER SERVING ||||||||||||||||||||||||||||||||||||||||||||||||||||||||||||||||||||||||||||||||||||||||||||||||||||||||
Calories 330 | Protein 19 g | Carbohydrate 33 g | Total fat 14 g
Sat fat 5 g | Fiber 4 g | Sodium 600 mg

Asparagus & Cheese Frittata

MAKES **6 SERVINGS**

12 lg. eggs

¾ c. grated Romano cheese

¾ tsp. salt

⅛ tsp. pepper

½ c. reduced-fat (2%) milk

1 Tbsp. olive oil

1 lb. asparagus, cut into
1-in. pieces

1 small bunch green onions,
thinly sliced

1. Preheat oven to 375°F. In medium bowl, with whisk, beat eggs, Romano, milk, ½ tsp. salt, and ⅛ tsp. pepper.

2. In nonstick 12-in. skillet with oven-safe handle, heat olive oil on medium-high. Stir in asparagus and ¼ tsp. salt; cook 4 min. Add green onions; cook 2 min., stirring often. Spread vegetable mixture evenly in skillet.

3. Reduce heat to medium-low. Pour egg mixture into skillet; cook 4 to 5 min., without stirring, until mixture starts to set around edge. Place skillet in oven; bake 9 to 10 min. or until set. Invert frittata onto serving plate; cut into wedges.

PER SERVING ‖‖

Calories 240 | Protein 18 g | Carbohydrate 5 g | Total fat 16 g
Sat fat 6 g | Fiber 2 g | Sodium 435 mg

Cheddar & Chicken Omelet

MAKES **1 SERVING**

¼ c. chopped onions

¼ c. chopped green peppers

1 oz. cooked chicken breast

¼ tsp. cumin

¼ tsp. oregano

Dash red pepper flakes

1 egg plus 2 egg whites

1 Tbsp. shredded Cheddar cheese

1 Tbsp. low-fat sour cream

1. Spray a microwave-proof cereal bowl with nonstick spray. Add the onions, green peppers, chicken, cumin, oregano and red pepper flakes, and stir. Microwave for 1½ min. Blot away excess moisture. Beat egg and egg whites, then stir into chicken mixture. Microwave for 1 min. Stir in Cheddar and microwave 1 min. more. Top with sour cream.

2. *Side for One:* 20 grapes.

PER SERVING ||||||||||||||||||||||||||||||||||||||||||||||||||||||||||||||||||||||||||||||||
Calories 290 | Protein 28 g | Carbohydrate 25 g | Total fat 11 g
Sat fat 5 g | Fiber 2 g | Sodium 290 mg

Morning Glory Muffins

MAKES **12 SERVINGS**

1¼ c. all-purpose flour

1 tsp. baking powder

½ tsp. baking soda

½ tsp. salt

½ tsp. ground cinnamon

1 c. old-fashioned or quick-cooking oats, uncooked

⅓ c. fat-free (skim) milk

⅔ c. unsweetened applesauce

¼ c. packed brown sugar

¼ c. light (mild) molasses

2 Tbsp. canola oil

1 lg. egg

3 med. carrots, shredded (about 1½ c.)

½ c. chopped dried plums (prunes)

1. Preheat oven to 400°F. Grease 12 standard muffin-pan cups, with baking spray, or line cups with fluted paper liners.

2. In large bowl, whisk together flour, baking powder, baking soda, salt and cinnamon; stir in oats. In medium bowl, with fork, mix milk, applesauce, sugar, molasses, oil and egg until blended; stir in carrots and prunes. Add apple-sauce mixture to flour mixture; stir just until flour is moistened (batter will be lumpy).

3. Spoon batter into prepared muffin-pan cups (muffin cups will be full). Bake 23 to 25 min. or until toothpick inserted in center of muffin comes out clean. Immediately remove muffins from pan. Serve muffins warm, or cool on wire rack to serve later.

Side for One: ½ c. plain nonfat Greek yogurt mixed with ½ tsp. honey and topped with 4 strawberries, sliced, and 2 tsp. each sliced almonds and unsweetened shredded coconut.

PER SERVING |||||||||||||||||||||||||||||||||||||||||||||||||||||||||||||||||||||||||||||
Calories 310 | Protein 17 g | Carbohydrate 44 g | Total fat 8 g
Sat fat 2.5 g | Fiber 4 g | Sodium 260 mg

Whole-Grain Pancakes

MAKES **12 PANCAKES, 6 SERVINGS**

1½ c. plain soy milk

⅔ c. quick-cooking oats

½ c. all-purpose flour

½ c. whole wheat flour

2 tsp. baking powder

¼ tsp. salt

3 tsp. canola oil

12 tsp. maple syrup

1. In medium bowl, combine soy milk and oats. Let stand 10 min.

2. Meanwhile, in large bowl, combine flours, baking powder and salt. Stir oil into oat mixture and add oat mixture to dry ingredients. Stir just until flour mixture is moistened (batter will be lumpy).

3. Spray 12-in. nonstick skillet with cooking spray; heat on medium 1 min. Pour batter by scant ¼ cups into skillet, making about 4 pancakes at a time. Cook until tops are bubbly, some bubbles burst and edges look dry. With wide spatula, turn pancakes and cook until undersides are golden. Transfer pancakes to platter. Cover; keep warm.

4. Repeat with remaining batter, using more nonstick cooking spray if necessary.

5. Place 2 pancakes on each plate and top each plate with 2 tsp. maple syrup

Side for One: 10 strawberries.

PER SERVING

Calories 280 | Protein 7 g | Carbohydrate 44 g | Total fat 9 g
Sat fat 0.5 g | Fiber 5 g | Sodium 280 mg

Lunches—about 500 calories

ASIAN TUNA SALAD

Mix 5 oz. canned water-packed tuna, drained, with ½ tsp. sesame oil and 1 tsp. reduced-sodium soy sauce. Top 2 c. baby spinach and ½ small-to-medium avocado, sliced, with tuna mixture; add 1 Tbsp. sliced almonds over salad. Serve with 4 Ak-Mak crackers.

PER SERVING | Calories 500 | Protein 44 g | Carbohydrate 36 g | Total fat 21 g | Sat fat 3 g Fiber 10 g | Sodium 690 mg

BLACK BEAN & CORN SALAD

Mix ½ c. reduced-sodium black beans, drained and rinsed, with ¼ c. canned or frozen corn (thawed, if frozen), ½ red pepper, chopped, 2 Tbsp. feta cheese, 1 tsp. olive oil and a squeeze of lime. Serve with 15 Food Should Taste Good multigrain tortilla chips. Have with 1 kiwifruit. PER SERVING | Calories 480 | Protein 14 g | Carbohydrate 64 g Total fat 10 g | Sat fat 3.5 g | Fiber 15 g | Sodium 780 mg

BURGER DAY

Toast a 100% whole wheat English muffin and spread with 1 oz. goat cheese; layer with 1 veggie burger, cooked according to package instructions, ½ jarred roasted red pepper and ⅛ small-to-medium avocado, sliced. Have with ½ red pepper, sliced, and 5 baby carrots dipped into ¼ c. hummus. PER SERVING | 490 Calories Protein 30 g | Carbohydrate 52 g | Total fat 20 g | Sat fat 6 g Fiber 13 g | Sodium 1,190 mg

BUTTERNUT SQUASH SOUP

Stir ½ chopped pear and 2 Tbsp. chopped, roasted almonds into 2 c. reduced-sodium butternut squash soup (such as Pacific; 90 calories per cup). Heat and top with 1 Tbsp. crumbled blue cheese. Serve with other pear half dusted with cinnamon and 1 whole wheat graham cracker rectangle. PER SERVING | Calories 480 Protein 11 g | Carbohydrate 76 g | Total fat 17 g | Sat fat 2.5 g | Fiber 14 g | Sodium 820 mg

CALIFORNIA CHICKEN SANDWICH

Between 2 slices of whole wheat bread (90 calories per slice) layer 1 Tbsp. light mayonnaise, 1 tsp. Dijon mustard, 2 oz. leftover grilled chicken or Applegate Natural Grilled Chicken Breast Strips, ¼ avocado and ¼ c. baby spinach. Serve with 10 SunChips and 1 apple. PER SERVING | Calories 530 | Protein 27 g | Carbohydrate 76 g | Total fat 15 g | Sat fat 1.5 g | Fiber 13 g | Sodium 690 mg

CHEESE PLATE

1 oz. each soft goat cheese, reduced-fat Cheddar Cheese and Brie, served with ¼ c. dried apricots, ½ apple, sliced, 1 Tbsp. walnut halves, 2 tsp. all-fruit preserves and 3 Ak-Mak crackers. PER SERVING | Calories 510 | Protein 23 g | Carbohydrate 54 g | Total fat 24 g | Sat fat 13 g | Fiber 6 g | Sodium 490 mg

CHICKEN, SPINACH & STRAWBERRY SALAD

Top 2 c. baby spinach with ⅔ c. shredded rotisserie chicken breast, ¼ c. strawberries, sliced, 2 Tbsp. each sliced almonds and feta crumbles, 1 tsp. red onion, chopped, and 2 Tbsp. reduced-fat balsamic vinaigrette. Serve with 6 Triscuits. PER SERVING | Calories 470 | Protein 39 g | Carbohydrate 33 g | Total fat 22 g | Sat fat 5 g | Fiber 8 g | Sodium 930 mg

CHICKEN SANDWICH

Spread 1 tsp. Dijon mustard over a whole wheat hamburger bun. Sandwich with ¼ c. cole slaw, 1 slice reduced-fat Swiss cheese and 3 oz. Applegate Natural Grilled Chicken Breast Strips. Serve with 6 baby carrots and 15 sweet potato chips. Have 1 orange for dessert. PER SERVING | Calories 50 | Protein 38 g | Carbohydrate 58 g | Total fat 17 g | Sat fat 3.5 g | Fiber 11 g | Sodium 750 mg

DIGIORNO

½ DiGiorno Tomato Mozzarella with Pesto Thin & Crispy Pizza
served with a salad made at home with 1 c. chopped romaine,
¼ c. cherry tomatoes, halved, ¼ med. avocado, sliced, 1 tsp. extra-
virgin olive oil and 2 tsp. balsamic vinegar. PER SERVING | Calories 500
Protein 20 g | Carbohydrate 62 g | Total fat 21 g | Sat fat 8 g | Fiber 5 g | Sodium 1,000 mg

EASY CAESAR SALAD

Top 2 c. chopped romaine with 3 oz. grilled chicken breast or
Applegate Natural Grilled Chicken Breast Strips, 2 Tbsp. Parmesan
cheese, and 1½ Tbsp. pine nuts. Drizzle with 2 Tbsp. Bolthouse
Farms Caesar Parmigiano Yogurt Dressing. Serve with a whole-
grain roll and 1 tsp. extra-virgin olive oil for dipping, and 1 c. fresh
cherries. PER SERVING | Calories 500 | Protein 36 g | Carbohydrate 45 g | Total fat 22 g
Sat fat 4 g | Fiber 7 g | Sodium 760 mg

GRAPEFRUIT & AVOCADO SALAD

Over 2 c. baby spinach, layer ½ grapefruit, sliced, and ½ avocado,
sliced. Top with ½ c. shredded chicken (from rotisserie or leftover
chicken breast) and 1 Tbsp. crumbled blue cheese. Drizzle with
1 tsp. extra-virgin olive oil and 2 tsp. balsamic vinegar. Serve with
1 whole wheat dinner roll. PER SERVING | Calories 510 | Protein 30 g
Carbohydrate 45 g | Total fat 26 g | Sat fat 5 g | Fiber 13 g | Sodium 390 mg

GREEK SALAD

Top 2 c. romaine lettuce with ¼ c. grape tomatoes, halved, ½ red
pepper, chopped, ½ c. reduced-sodium chickpeas, drained and
rinsed, and 2 Tbsp. feta crumbles. Sprinkle with ½ tsp. oregano,
2 tsp. olive oil, and 1 tsp. red wine vinegar. Serve with large
(6½-in.) whole wheat pita. PER SERVING | Calories 480 | Protein 18 g
Carbohydrate 67 g | Total fat 16 g | Sat fat 4.5 g | Fiber 13 g | Sodium 590 mg

GREEK GRAIN SALAD

To 1 c. cooked quinoa, add ½ c. reduced-sodium chickpeas, rinsed, ¼ each cucumber and red pepper, chopped, ½ c. cherry tomatoes, halved, 1 tsp. pine nuts and 2 Tbsp. feta cheese crumbles. Mix in 1 tsp. olive oil and 1 tsp. red wine vinegar. PER SERVING | Calories 500

Protein 20 g | Carbohydrate 71 g | Total fat 15 g | Sat fat 3.5 g | Fiber 13 g | Sodium 260 mg

MEDITERRANEAN GRILLED CHEESE

Sandwich 2 oz. part-skim mozzarella, 3 tomato slices and 1 c. baby spinach between 2 slices whole wheat bread. Brush 2 tsp. extra-virgin olive oil on the outside bread halves. Cook in a nonstick skillet, flipping halfway through, until mozzarella melts. Serve with 1 c. vegetable juice chilled or heated in microwave (like soup). Have 2 kiwifruit for dessert. PER SERVING | Calories 490 | Protein 25 g

Carbohydrate 60 g | Total fat 17 g | Sat fat 7 g | Fiber 12 g | Sodium 1,140 mg

MEDITERRANEAN WRAP

In a 100-calorie whole wheat tortilla (such as La Tortilla Factory), spread ¼ c. hummus, 2 Tbsp. reduced-fat feta, ¼ c. grated carrots, ¼ cucumber, sliced, 3 tomato slices and 1 c. baby spinach. Serve with 1½ c. grapes. PER SERVING | Calories 484 | Protein 21 g | Carbohydrate 88 g

Total fat 12 g | Sat fat 2.5 g | Fiber 16 g | Sodium 920 mg

NACHOS

Spread 15 Food Should Taste Good multigrain tortilla chips over a microwavable plate and top with ¼ c. reduced-fat Mexican or Cheddar cheese shreds. Heat for 30 sec. or until cheese melts. Meanwhile, heat ½ c. vegetarian refried beans and chop ½ red pepper. Top chips with warm beans and red pepper chunks, and serve with 2 Tbsp. guacamole. PER SERVING | Calories 500 | Protein 19 g

Carbohydrate 56 g | Total fat 13 g | Sat fat 4.5 g | Fiber 15 g | Sodium 1,080 mg

NUT BUTTER SANDWICH

Spread 2 Tbsp. almond butter over 2 pieces 100% whole wheat bread and layer with ¼ c. strawberries, sliced. Have with another cup of strawberries served with a dip made from 2 Tbsp. plain nonfat Greek yogurt and 1 tsp. honey. PER SERVING | Calories 480

Protein 17 g | Carbohydrate 60 g | Total fat 21 g | Sat fat 2 g | Fiber 9 g | Sodium 420 mg

PANERA BREAD TAKEOUT

½ Mediterranean Veggie Café Sandwich on XL Tomato Basil Loaf with 1 c. Low-Fat Garden Vegetable Soup with Pesto and 1 apple.

PER SERVING | Calories 480 | Protein 14 g | Carbohydrate 91 g | Total fat 11 g | Sat fat 2 g

Fiber 11 g | Sodium 1,310 mg

SOUPER SOUP

Heat 2 c. boxed mushroom soup (such as Imagine; 80 calories per cup) with ½ c. frozen brown rice, cooked, ½ c. canned lentil beans and 1 c. baby spinach until spinach wilts and soup is warm throughout. Dessert: 1 pear. PER SERVING | Calories 480 | Protein 20 g

Carbohydrate 89 g | Total fat 7 g | Sat fat 0 g | Fiber 21 g | Sodium 820 mg

SPINACH SALAD PITA

Mix 2 c. baby spinach with 2 tsp. dried cranberries, 2 Tbsp. blue cheese crumbles, 2 Tbsp. sliced almonds, 2 tsp. extra-virgin olive oil and 2 tsp. balsamic vinegar. Stuff salad mixture and 2 oz. grilled chicken breast or Applegate Natural Grilled Chicken Breast Strips into a large (6½-in.) whole wheat pita. PER SERVING | Calories 490

Protein 30 g | Carbohydrate 49 g | Total fat 22 g | Sat fat 5 g | Fiber 9 g | Sodium 850 mg

TUNA BEAN SALAD

Mix one 5 oz. can tuna, in water, with ¼ c. cannellini beans and ¼ c. sun-dried tomatoes (jarred in oil). Top 2 c. baby spinach with ¼ avocado, sliced, and tuna mixture. Serve with 2 Ak-Mak crackers. **PER SERVING** | Calories 490 | Protein 43 g | Carbohydrate 44 g | Total fat 16 g | Sat fat 2.5 g | Fiber 13 g | Sodium 500 mg

Dinners—about 500 calories

Beef & Bulgur Falafel

MAKES **4 SERVINGS**

¾ c. bulgur wheat

8 oz. lean ground beef

2 scallions, sliced

2 cloves garlic, finely chopped

1 tsp. ground cumin

1 tsp. ground turmeric

Kosher salt

1 Tbsp. olive oil

¾ c. fresh mint leaves, chopped

1 c. plain fat-free yogurt

½ cucumber, diced

4 multigrain pitas, halved

¼ sm. red cabbage, shredded (1½ c.)

1 lg. yellow pepper, sliced

1. Bring pot of water to a boil. Place bulgur in medium bowl. Add boiling water to cover. Soak until tender, 15 to 20 min. Drain bulgur.

2. Heat oven to 425°F. Line rimmed baking sheet with foil. Mix beef, scallions, garlic, cumin, turmeric, ¼ tsp. salt and bulgur in a bowl.

3. Form mixture into 24 ½-in.-thick patties and place on prepared sheet. Brush with oil and roast until cooked through, 8 to 10 min.

4. Mix ¼ c. mint, yogurt and cucumber in a bowl.

5. Fill pita with cabbage, yellow pepper and remaining mint. Add patties, top with yogurt sauce.

Side for One: 1 serving Spinach Sauté (see page 289) topped with 1 tsp. pine nuts.

PER SERVING

Calories 480 | Protein 27 g | Carbohydrate 74 g | Total fat 12 g | Sat fat 2 g | Fiber 15 g | Sodium 620 mg

Black Bean Soup

MAKES **6 SERVINGS**

2 Tbsp. olive oil

1 lg. onion, diced

1 green bell pepper, seeded and divided

2 lg. plum tomatoes, seeded and chopped

4 cloves garlic, crushed

1½ tsp. dried oregano

1½ tsp. ground cumin

1 dried bay leaf

3 (19-oz.) cans black beans, rinsed and drained

5 c. reduced-sodium chicken stock or broth

1 c. frozen whole-kernel corn

1 c. diced smoked ham

¼ c. chopped cilantro

1 tsp. hot red-pepper sauce, or to taste

Reduced-fat sour cream, for garnish

Cilantro sprigs, for garnish

Lime wedges, for garnish

1. Heat oil in a 5-qt. soup pot over medium-high heat; add onion, bell pepper and tomatoes. Sauté 10 min. or until onions and peppers have softened. Stir in garlic, oregano, cumin and bay leaf, then stir in beans and cook 2 min., stirring constantly. Add stock and bring to a boil; reduce heat to medium-low, cover and simmer 20 min.

2. Using a stick blender, puree soup until about half the black beans are pureed (or, if using a regular blender, puree half the soup). Stir in corn, ham, cilantro and hot-pepper sauce. Cook over medium heat 3 to 4 min. longer, until corn and ham are heated through.

3. Ladle into bowls. Garnish with 1 Tbsp. reduced-fat sour cream, cilantro sprigs and a squeeze of lime, if desired.

Side for One: 5 Food Should Taste Good multigrain chips.

PER SERVING

Calories 480 | Protein 26 g | Carbohydrate 57 g | Total fat 11 g
Sat fat 2.5 g | Fiber 18 g | Sodium 980 mg

Bulgur Pilaf with Garbanzos & Dried Apricots

MAKES **4 SERVINGS (AS A MAIN DISH)**

1 (14- to 14½-oz.) can
  vegetable or chicken broth

1 c. bulgur

1 Tbsp. olive oil

1 sm. onion, chopped

2 tsp. curry powder

1 clove garlic, crushed with
  press

1 (15- to 19-oz.) can
  garbanzo beans
  (chickpeas), rinsed
  and drained

½ c. dried apricots, chopped

½ tsp. salt

¼ c. (loosely packed) fresh
  parsley leaves, chopped

1. In 2-qt. covered saucepan, heat ¾ c. water and 1¼ c. broth to boiling on high. Stir in bulgur; heat to boiling. Reduce heat to medium-low; cover and simmer 12 to 15 min. or until liquid is absorbed. Remove saucepan from heat. Uncover and fluff bulgur with fork to separate grains.

2. Meanwhile, in 12-in. nonstick skillet, heat oil on medium 1 min. Add onion and cook 10 minutes, stirring occasionally. Stir in curry powder and garlic; cook 1 min.

3. Stir in garbanzo beans, apricots, salt and remaining ½ c. vegetable broth; heat to boiling. Remove saucepan from heat; stir in bulgur and parsley.

Side for One: 2 c. baby spinach sautéed in 1 tsp. extra-virgin olive oil until the leaves are wilted.

PER SERVING ||||||||||||||||||||||||||||||||||||||||||||||||||||||||||||||||||||||||||||||||||||||||||
Calories 500 | Protein 14 g | Carbohydrate 71 g | Total fat 19 g
Sat fat 2 g | Fiber 16 g | Sodium 460 mg

Buttermilk Oven-Fried Chicken Tenders

MAKES **4 SERVINGS**

1½ lbs. skinless chicken breast

⅔ c. reduced-fat buttermilk

½ tsp. paprika

⅔ c. Fiber One Original cereal

⅓ c. panko bread crumbs

2 Tbsp. onion soup mix

Salt and pepper to taste

Nonstick cooking spray

1. Wash and pat dry chicken and cut into 24 strips. Put in large sealable container or plastic bag. Add buttermilk and paprika, and mix well into chicken. Seal and refrigerate for at least 1 hr.

2. Using blender or food processor, grind cereal to consistency of bread crumbs. Pour into large bowl. Add panko and onion soup mix. Season lightly with salt and pepper.

3. Remove chicken pieces from bag, giving each a good shake to remove excess buttermilk. Spray large baking sheet with nonstick spray. Bake in a preheated 375°F oven for 10 min. Turn with a spatula and return to oven for an additional 10 min. or until chicken is crunchy.

Side for One: 1 serving Butternut Squash Fries (page 281).

Dessert for One: 1 Apple Crisp (page 290).

PER SERVING ||||||||||||||||||||||||||||||||||||||||||||||||||||||||||||||||||||||||||||||||||||||||||
Calories 520 | Protein 48 g | Carbohydrate 80 g | Total fat 6 g
Sat fat 1.5 g | Fiber 14 g | Sodium 730 mg

Chicken & Mushrooms with Brown Rice

MAKES **4 MAIN DISH SERVINGS**

2 Tbsp. olive oil

1¼ lbs. skinless, boneless chicken thighs

1 (10-oz.) pkg. sliced cremini mushrooms

2 med. stalks celery, thinly sliced

1 tsp. chopped fresh thyme leaves

1 (14- to 14½-oz.) can chicken broth

1 c. instant brown rice

½ c. dry white wine

¼ tsp. salt

¼ tsp. coarsely ground black pepper

8 baby summer squash, halved and steamed

1. In 12-in. skillet, heat oil on medium-high until hot. Add chicken and cook, covered, 5 min. Reduce heat to medium; turn chicken and cook, covered, 5 min. more. Transfer to plate.

2. To same skillet, add mushrooms, celery and thyme; cook 5 min. or until vegetables are softened, stirring occasionally. Add broth, rice, wine, salt and pepper; heat to boiling.

3. Return chicken to skillet. Reduce heat to low; cover and simmer about 12 min. or until juices run clear when thickest part of chicken is pierced with knife, and rice is cooked.

4. Serve with steamed squash.

Dessert: Buttermilk Panna Cotta (page 292).

PER SERVING ||||||||||||||||||||||||||||||||||||||||||||||||||||||||||||||||||||||||||||||||||
Calories 500 | Protein 39 g | Carbohydrate 45 g | Total fat 16 g
Sat fat 3.5 g | Fiber 6 g | Sodium 790 mg

Chicken with Arugula Pesto Spaghetti

MAKES **4 SERVINGS**

1 lb. cherry tomatoes

1 tsp. kosher salt

½ tsp. freshly ground pepper

4 oz. whole wheat spaghetti

4 (3-oz.) skinless, boneless chicken-breast halves

2 c. baby arugula

1 c. fresh basil leaves

½ c. grated fresh Parmesan cheese

⅓ c. pine nuts

⅓ c. olive oil

1. Preheat oven to 450°F. Preheat large ridged grill pan.

2. Place tomatoes on baking sheet lined with parchment or foil; lightly coat with olive oil cooking spray, and season with ¼ tsp. salt and ¼ tsp. pepper. Roast tomatoes 10 to 12 min., or until lightly charred and softened.

3. Cook spaghetti according to package directions.

4. Meanwhile, lightly coat chicken breasts with cooking spray and season with ¼ tsp. salt and remaining pepper. Place chicken on hot grill. Cook 4 min. per side, or until just cooked through. Remove to plate; tent with foil and let rest.

5. In food processor, combine arugula, basil, Parmesan, pine nuts, oil, ¼ c. water and remaining salt. Pulse until smooth. (Makes 1¼ cups pesto.) Combine pesto with spaghetti.

6. Divide spaghetti among 4 plates. Place chicken over pasta. Serve with roasted tomatoes.

PER SERVING |||||||||||||||||||||||||||||||||||||||||||||||||||||||||||||||||||||||||||||||||||||||||||||
Calories 500 | Protein 30 g | Carbohydrate 27 g | Total fat 31 g
Sat fat 5 g | Fiber 16 g | Sodium 360 mg

Chicken Salad with Orzo & Feta

MAKES **4 SERVINGS**

1 lemon

1 pt. cherry tomatoes, cut in half

1 med. orange pepper (8 oz.), chopped

3 cloves garlic, crushed with press

2 Tbsp. extra-virgin olive oil

¼ tsp. dried oregano

Salt and pepper

1 lb. skinless, boneless chicken breasts, cut into 1-in. chunks

1 c. whole wheat orzo pasta

4 stalks celery, thinly sliced at an angle

2 oz. feta cheese, crumbled (½ c.)

¼ c. walnuts, crushed

1. Preheat oven to 450°F. Heat 4-qt. saucepan of water to boiling on high. From lemon, finely grate 1 tsp. peel and squeeze 2 Tbsp. juice.

2. On one side of 18" by 12" rimmed baking sheet, toss tomatoes and orange pepper with garlic, 1 Tbsp. oil and ⅛ tsp. each oregano, salt and freshly ground black pepper. Spread in even layer. On other side of pan, toss chicken with lemon peel, 1 Tbsp. oil and ⅛ tsp. each oregano, salt and freshly ground black pepper. Spread in even layer. Roast 13 min. or until chicken loses pink color throughout (165°F).

3. While chicken and vegetables roast, cook orzo according to package directions. Drain well and transfer to large bowl. Add chicken and vegetables, with their juices, to orzo, along with celery and lemon juice. Toss until well mixed. Top with feta and walnuts.

Dessert for One: 25 grapes.

PER SERVING ||||||||||||||||||||||||||||||||||||||||||||||||||||||||||||||||||||||||||||||

Calories 509 | Protein 37 g | Carbohydrate 54 g | Total fat 17 g
Sat fat 4 g | Fiber 8 g | Sodium 300 mg

Classic Minestrone

MAKES **4 SERVINGS**

1 c. pearl barley

1 Tbsp. olive oil

2 c. green cabbage, thinly sliced (about ¼ small head)

2 lg. carrots, each cut lengthwise in half, then crosswise into ½-in.-thick slices

2 lg. celery stalks, cut into ½-in. dice

1 med. onion, cut into ½-in. dice

1 clove garlic, finely chopped

2 (14½-oz.) cans vegetable broth (3½ c.)

1 (14½-oz.) can diced tomatoes

Salt

1 med. (about 6 oz.) zucchini, cut into ½-in. dice

½ lb. green beans, cut into ½-in. pieces (about 1 c.)

Light Pesto

1 c. fresh basil leaves, firmly packed

2 Tbsp. olive oil

Salt

¼ c. Romano cheese, freshly grated

1 clove garlic, finely chopped

1. Heat 5- to 6-qt. Dutch oven over medium-high heat until hot. Add barley and cook 3 to 4 min. or until toasted and fragrant, stirring constantly. Transfer barley to small bowl; set aside.

2. In same Dutch oven, heat oil over medium-high heat until hot. Add cabbage, carrots, celery and onion; cook 8 to 10 min. or until vegetables are tender and lightly browned, stirring occasionally. Add garlic and cook 30 sec. or until fragrant. Stir in barley, 3 c. water, broth, tomatoes and ¼ tsp. salt. Cover and heat to boiling over high heat. Reduce heat to low and simmer, covered, 25 min.

3. Stir zucchini and beans into Dutch oven; increase heat to medium and cook, covered, 10 to 15 min. or until all vegetables and barley are tender.

4. In blender container with narrow base or mini food processor, combine basil, oil, 2 Tbsp. water and ¼ tsp. salt; cover and blend until pureed. Transfer pesto to small bowl; stir in Romano and garlic. Makes about ½ c. pesto.

5. Ladle minestrone into 4 large soup bowls. Top each serving with some pesto.

Side for One: 1 whole wheat dinner roll.

PER SERVING ||||||||||||||||||||||||||||||||||||||||||||||||||||||||||||||||||||||||||||||||

Calories 500 | Protein 14 g | Carbohydrate 78 g | Total fat 15 g

Sat fat 3 g | Fiber 18 g | Sodium 990 mg

Feta Turkey Burgers with Yogurt Mint Sauce

MAKES **4 SERVINGS**

½ c. plus 2 Tbsp. plain fat-free yogurt

2 green onions, green and white parts separated and thinly sliced

½ c. fresh mint leaves, finely chopped

1 lb. lean ground turkey

1½ oz. feta cheese, finely crumbled

1½ tsp. ground coriander

Salt and pepper

4 burger rolls

2 tomatoes, thinly sliced

1. Preheat an outdoor grill for covered direct grilling on medium.

2. In small bowl, combine ½ c. yogurt, white parts of green onions and half the chopped mint.

3. In bowl, with hands, combine ground turkey, feta, coriander, ⅛ tsp. salt, ½ tsp. freshly ground black pepper, green parts of green onions, and remaining mint and yogurt. Mix well, then form into 4½-in.-round patties (each ¾ in. thick).

4. Place turkey patties on hot grill; cover and cook 12 to 13 min. or just until turkey loses its pink color throughout, turning once. (Burgers should reach an internal temperature of 165°F.) During last 2 min. of cooking, add rolls to grill. Cook 2 min., or until warmed, turning once.

5. Put turkey burgers on rolls. Top with tomato and yogurt sauce.

Side for One: 1 c. boxed mushroom soup (such as Imagine) and 10 sweet potato fries.

PER SERVING ||||||||||||||||||||||||||||||||||||||||||||||||||||||||||||||||||||||||||||||||||||||||||||||

Calories 510 | Protein 42 g | Carbohydrate 59 g | Total fat 14 g
Sat fat 2.5 g | Fiber 7 g | Sodium 870 mg

Greek Chicken

MAKES **4 SERVINGS**

4 boneless, skinless chicken breasts, cut into 1-in. pieces

Kosher salt

Freshly ground pepper

2 Tbsp. olive oil

2 c. marinara sauce

½ c. Kalamata olives, pitted and halved

2 Tbsp. chopped fresh parsley

2 oz. feta cheese, crumbled

1. Season chicken with kosher salt and freshly ground pepper. In a large skillet, heat oil over medium heat. Add chicken and cook about 5 min., until lightly browned all over.

2. Pour in marinara sauce and olives, reduce heat to low, and cook until heated through. Sprinkle with parsley and feta.

Side for One: Roasted asparagus (see box on page 287) and ½ c. cooked whole wheat orzo.

PER SERVING |||||||||||||||||||||||||||||||||||||||||||||||||||||||||||||||||||||||||||||||||||||||

Calories 500 | Protein 38 g | Carbohydrate 40 g | Total fat 21 g

Sat fat 5 g | Fiber 10 g | Sodium 900 mg

Greek-Style Stuffed Peppers

MAKES **8 SERVINGS**

8 lg. red, yellow, orange and/or green peppers, with stems if possible

2 (14½-oz.) cans chicken broth

1½ c. bulgur

1 Tbsp. olive oil

1 med. onion, chopped

3 cloves garlic, crushed with press

1 lb. lean (90%) ground beef

1 pkg. (10-oz.) frozen chopped spinach, thawed and squeezed dry

½ c. loosely packed fresh dill, chopped

2 (28-oz.) cans crushed tomatoes

1 c. crumbled feta cheese (4 oz.)

Salt and pepper

1. Slice off top of each pepper; reserve. Remove seeds and ribs, and slice bottom of each pepper so it will stand upright.

2. Arrange peppers and tops on microwave-safe plate. Cook, uncovered, in microwave on High 4 min. With tongs, transfer tops to paper towel. Microwave peppers 4 to 5 min. longer or until just tender. Invert peppers onto paper towels to drain.

3. In microwave-safe bowl, combine chicken broth and bulgur. Cook, uncovered, in microwave on High 12 to 15 min. or until most of broth is absorbed.

4. Meanwhile, in deep 12-in. skillet, heat oil on medium until hot. Stirring frequently, cook onion and garlic 5 min., until onion turns golden. Remove ¼ c. onion mixture. Add beef to remaining onion in skillet and cook 6 to 8 min. or until beef is no longer pink. Remove from heat.

5. Preheat oven to 350°F. In skillet, mix beef, bulgur, spinach, dill, 1 c. tomatoes, and ¾ c. feta. Fill peppers with bulgur mixture; sprinkle with remaining feta.

continued on next page

continued from previous page

6. Replace pepper tops.

7. Wipe skillet clean. In same skillet, combine remaining tomatoes, reserved onion mixture, ¼ tsp. salt and ¼ tsp. freshly ground black pepper; heat to boiling on medium-high.

8. Divide tomato sauce between two 8" by 8" glass baking dishes. Place 4 peppers in each dish. Cover with foil and bake 35 min.

Side for One: 1 serving Roasted Beet & Olive Salad with Orange & Mint (page 286).

Dessert for One: 1 serving Chocolate Pudding Cake (page 293)

PER SERVING ||||||||||||||||||||||||||||||||||||||||||||||||||||||||||||||||||||||||||||||||||||||||||||||||
Calories 500 | Protein 25 g | Carbohydrate 70 g | Total fat 17 g
Sat fat 5 g | Fiber 15g | Sodium 1,450 mg

Grilled Portobello Burgers with Pesto Mayo

MAKES **4 SERVINGS**

1½ Tbsp. extra-virgin olive oil

1 tsp. garlic paste, or half that amount pressed fresh garlic

¼ tsp. kosher salt

¼ tsp. black pepper

4 (4-in.) portobello mushrooms, stems removed, gills scraped from beneath caps

2 Tbsp. basil pesto

2 Tbsp. reduced-fat olive oil mayonnaise (such as Kraft)

1 tsp. fresh lemon juice

8 (¼-in.-thick) slices fresh mozzarella cheese

4 sandwich-size whole wheat English muffins, split and toasted

4 butter-leaf lettuce leaves

2 jarred roasted bell peppers, quartered

1. Heat an outdoor grill with a medium-hot fire, or heat a stovetop grill pan over medium heat. Combine olive oil, garlic paste, salt and pepper; lightly brush mixture over mushrooms.

2. Stir pesto, mayonnaise and lemon juice in a bowl until smooth.

3. Grill mushroom caps about 3 min. per side, until tender, placing 2 slices of cheese on top of each mushroom during the last minute of grilling.

4. Spread cut sides of muffins with pesto mixture. Line muffin bottoms with lettuce leaves. Place mushrooms over lettuce, then top with roasted peppers and muffin tops.

Dessert for One: 1 c. watermelon chunks.

PER SERVING ||||||||||||||||||||||||||||||||||||||||||||||||||||||||||||||||||||||||||||||||||||||||||||||
Calories 480 | Protein 23 g | Carbohydrate 38 g | Total fat 27 g
Sat fat 9 g | Fiber 5 g | Sodium 760 mg

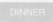

Grilled Swordfish Kebabs with Parsley-Olive Salsa

MAKES **4 SERVINGS**

Parsley-Olive Salsa

¼ c. flat-leaf parsley, chopped

8 pitted oil-cured olives, chopped

4 oil-packed sun-dried tomato halves, drained and diced

1 tsp. garlic paste

2 Tbsp. extra-virgin olive oil

2 Tbsp. water

½ tsp. grated lemon zest

2 Tbsp. lemon juice

¼ tsp. crushed red pepper flakes

Kebabs

1 red onion, cut into 20 wedges

1½ lbs. (1-in.-thick) swordfish or halibut, skin removed, cut into 20 chunks

20 mixed baby bell peppers (or 20 pieces of cut-up bell peppers)

Olive oil cooking spray

½ tsp. kosher salt

½ tsp. freshly ground white or black pepper

1. *Salsa:* Combine all ingredients in a bowl.

2. *Kebabs:* Heat a stovetop grill pan over medium heat. Alternately thread onto four 12-in. metal skewers 5 onion pieces, swordfish pieces and bell peppers. Spray kebabs with olive oil cooking spray, and season with salt and pepper.

3. Grill kebabs 8 to 10 min., turning skewers every 2 min., until swordfish is just barely opaque and vegetables are lightly charred. Spoon salsa over kebabs.

Side for One: Cook ½ c. whole wheat couscous according to package directions. Toss with 1 Tbsp. sun-dried tomatoes, jarred in oil and drained, and 1 Tbsp. pine nuts.

PER SERVING

Calories 490 | Protein 40 g | Carbohydrate 32 g | Total fat 23 g
Sat fat 3.5 g | Fiber 6 g | Sodium 510 mg

Halibut with Tomato, Olive & Pine Nut Relish

MAKES **4 SERVINGS**

3 Tbsp. pine nuts

½ c. pitted Kalamata olives, cut in slivers

½ c. pitted green olives, cut in slivers

½ c. finely diced red tomato

½ c. finely diced yellow tomato

1 small shallot, minced

½ tsp. grated lemon zest

1 Tbsp. lemon juice

3 Tbsp. extra-virgin olive oil

2 Tbsp. chopped chervil or parsley

Freshly ground pepper, to taste

4 (6-oz., 1-in. thick) halibut fillets without skin

Flour, for dusting

½ tsp. kosher salt

1. Toast pine nuts in a dry, nonstick skillet over medium heat 3 to 4 min., tossing frequently, until lightly toasted; remove to a small cup.

2. In a medium bowl, combine olives, tomatoes, shallot, lemon zest and juice, and 1 Tbsp. oil; toss. Stir in chervil and freshly ground pepper.

3. Dust fillets in flour, tapping off excess; season with salt and a few grindings of pepper. Heat the remaining 2 Tbsp. oil in a nonstick skillet over medium-high heat; add fillets. Cook 6 min.; turn fillets and continue to cook 4 min. longer, or until just barely opaque in thickest parts. Transfer to plates and spoon relish over fillets. Garnish with pine nuts.

Side for One: 2 c. baby spinach, steamed and squirted with lemon juice; ½ c. cooked quinoa.

PER SERVING |||||||||||||||||||||||||||||||||||||||||||||||||||||||||||||||||||||||||||||||||||||
Calories 520 | Protein 42 g | Carbohydrate 32 g | Total fat 25 g
Sat fat 2.5 g | Fiber 6 g | Sodium 900 mg

Hoisin-Glazed Salmon

MAKES **4 SERVINGS**

3 Tbsp. hoisin sauce

¼ tsp. Chinese five-spice powder

4 (6-oz.) pieces skinless salmon fillet

1 c. quinoa

1 Tbsp. rice vinegar

1 Tbsp. reduced-sodium soy sauce

1 bunch radishes, trimmed and thinly sliced

2 green onions, thinly sliced

1. Preheat oven to 400°F. In small bowl, combine hoisin and five-spice powder. In 13" by 9" glass or ceramic baking dish, place salmon, flat side down. Spread hoisin mixture on top of salmon. Bake salmon 15 to 17 min. or until opaque throughout.

2. Meanwhile, in 12-in. skillet, toast quinoa on medium 5 min. or until fragrant and golden, stirring frequently.

3. Stir 2 c. water into toasted quinoa; heat to boiling on high. Reduce heat to low; cover and simmer 15 min. or until water is absorbed. Remove skillet from heat and stir in vinegar, soy sauce, radishes and green onions until blended.

PER SERVING ||||||||||||||||||||||||||||||||||||||||||||||||||||||||||||||||||||||||||||||||||||||||||
Calories 500 | Protein 41 g | Carbohydrate 36 g | Total fat 21 g
Sat fat 6 g | Fiber 4 g | Sodium 570 mg

Italian Steak Kebabs over Orzo

MAKES **4 SERVINGS**

12 baby pattypan squash or
3 or 4 zucchini cut into
1½-in. chunks

1 lb. beef tenderloin, cut into
12 1½-in. chunks

1 lg. orange bell pepper,
seeded and cut into
12 chunks

12 sm. white mushrooms

½ c. low-fat Caesar salad
dressing

2 c. hot steamed orzo

1. Blanch squash in salted boiling water for
2 min. Drain and rinse under cold water. Pat dry.

2. In large bowl, mix squash, beef, bell pepper,
mushrooms and dressing. Marinate 15 min.
Thread meat and vegetables onto skewers. Grill
or broil for 8 to 10 min. for medium-rare, turning
several times. Serve over orzo.

Dessert for One: 1 serving Fire-Roasted
Nectarines with Berry Salsa (page 294).

PER SERVING ||||||||||||||||||||||||||||||||||||||||||||||||||||||||||||||||||||||||||||||||
Calories 470 | Protein 33 g | Carbohydrate 76 g | Total fat 7 g
Sat fat 2 g | Fiber 9 g | Sodium 400 mg

Lamb Lollichops with Wine Sauce

MAKES **4 SERVINGS**

1 Tbsp. olive oil

5 cloves garlic, peeled

5 sprigs fresh rosemary

8 rib lamb chops, 1 in. thick (about 2 lb.), well trimmed

Kosher salt and pepper

1 c. red wine

1. In large skillet on medium-high, heat oil, garlic and rosemary. Cook 1 min., stirring constantly, to season and prepare pan; then discard oil, garlic and herbs.

2. Sprinkle lamb chops with ½ tsp. kosher salt and ¼ tsp. freshly ground black pepper. Place in same skillet and cook 3 to 4 min. per side, or until medium rare. Transfer to platter and cover to keep warm.

3. Pour off pan drippings. Increase heat to high, add wine to pan and stir about 3 min., scraping up brown bits, until liquid is reduced to ½ c. To serve, place 2 lamb chops on each plate and drizzle with sauce.

Side for One: 1 serving Spinach Sauté (page 289).

Dessert for One: 1 clementine.

PER SERVING ||||||||||||||||||||||||||||||||||||||||||||||||||||||||||||||||||||||||||||||||||||||||||||||||

Calories 490 | Protein 49 g | Carbohydrate 20 g | Total fat 19 g
Sat fat 7 g | Fiber 5 g | Sodium 380 mg

Lemon Oregano Roasted Chicken

MAKES **6 SERVINGS**

3 lemons

¼ c. loosely packed fresh oregano leaves, chopped

¼ c. loosely packed fresh parsley leaves, chopped

1 Tbsp. olive oil

Salt and ground black pepper

1 chicken (about 3½ lbs.), cut into quarters and skin removed from all but wings

1. Preheat oven to 450°F. Line rimmed pastry sheet with foil. From 2 lemons, grate 1 Tbsp. peel and squeeze 3 Tbsp. juice. Cut lemon into wedges; set aside.

2. In large bowl, combine lemon peel and juice, oregano, parsley, oil, 1 tsp. salt and ¼ tsp. pepper. Add chicken; toss to coat. Arrange chicken in prepared pan.

3. Roast chicken, without turning, 30 to 35 min. or until juices run clear when thickest part of chicken is pierced with tip of knife. Transfer to warm platter. Serve with lemon wedges to squeeze over chicken.

Side for One: Roasted Sweet Potatoes (page 288)

PER SERVING ||||||||||||||||||||||||||||||||||||||||||||||||||||||||||||||||||||||||||||||||||||
Calories 480 | Protein 56 g | Carbohydrate 33 g | Total fat 12 g
Sat fat 2.5 g | Fiber 6 g | Sodium 280 mg

Moroccan-Style Chickpea & Sweet Potato Stew

MAKES **4 SERVINGS**

2 tsp. olive oil

1 med. onion, chopped

3 cloves garlic, crushed with press

1½ tsp. curry powder

1½ tsp. ground cumin

¼ tsp. ground allspice

1 (14½-oz.) can diced tomatoes

1 (14- to 14½-oz.) can reduced-sodium chicken broth

1 c. garbanzo beans (chickpeas), rinsed and drained

1 lg. sweet potato (1 lb.), peeled and cut into ¾-in. chunks

1 zucchini (12 oz.), thickly sliced

1 c. whole-grain couscous

2 Tbsp. chopped fresh mint leaves

1. In 12-in. skillet, heat oil on medium. Add onion and cook 8 to 10 min. or until tender and lightly browned, stirring occasionally. Stir in garlic, curry powder, cumin and allspice; cook 30 sec.

2. To onion mixture in skillet, add tomatoes, broth, beans and sweet potato; cover and heat to boiling on medium-high. Reduce heat to medium; cover and cook 10 min. Stir in zucchini and cook, covered, 10 min. or until all vegetables are tender.

3. Meanwhile, prepare couscous according to package instructions.

4. Stir chopped mint into stew. Spoon stew over couscous to serve.

Dessert for One: 1 serving Brandy-Poached Winter Fruit with Cinnamon & Star Anise (page 291).

PER SERVING
Calories 480 | Protein 15 g | Carbohydrate 97 g | Total fat 4 g
Sat fat 0 g | Fiber 5 g | Sodium 710 mg

Pasta with Goat Cheese & Walnuts

MAKES **6 SERVINGS**

½ c. walnuts, chopped

2 cloves garlic, chopped

1 Tbsp. extra-virgin olive oil

⅝ tsp. freshly ground pepper

1 box (13.25 oz.) med. whole-grain shells

1 lb. frozen peas

6 oz. goat cheese, softened

2⅜ tsp. salt

1. Heat covered 6-qt. pot of water to boiling on high. Add 2 tsp. salt.

2. In 8- to 10-in. skillet, combine walnuts, garlic and oil. Cook on medium until golden and fragrant, stirring occasionally. Stir in ⅛ tsp. each salt and freshly ground black pepper.

3. Add pasta to boiling water in pot. Cook 1 min. less than minimum time that package directs, stirring occasionally. Add peas; cook 1 min. longer. Reserve 1 c. pasta cooking water. Drain pasta and peas; return to pot. Add goat cheese, ½ c. cooking water, ¼ tsp. salt and ½ tsp. freshly ground black pepper. If mixture is dry, toss with additional cooking water. To serve, top with garlic-and-walnut mixture.

Side for One: Roasted Broccoli (page 287)

PER SERVING ||||||||||||||||||||||||||||||||||||||||||||||||||||||||||||||||||||||||||||||||||||
Calories 520 | Protein 23 g | Carbohydrate 67 g | Total fat 19 g
Sat fat 5 g | Fiber 14 g | Sodium 160 mg

Penne with Escarole, White Beans & Toasted Bread Crumbs

MAKES **6 SERVINGS**

½ c. dried plain bread crumbs

5 Tbsp. olive oil

1 lb. dried whole wheat penne or cut ziti pasta

5 anchovy fillets, minced

2 cloves garlic, finely chopped

1 head escarole (1½ lbs.), separated into leaves, torn into 2-in. pieces and washed well (keep leaves wet)

1 (15.5-oz.) can cannellini beans, drained and rinsed

¼ tsp. kosher salt

¼ tsp. ground black pepper

1. Bring a large pot of salted water to a boil.

2. Toast bread crumbs in a dry nonstick skillet over medium-high heat for 3 min., stirring constantly until well browned. Stir in 1 Tbsp. oil until crumbs are moistened; transfer crumbs to a small cup and reserve.

3. Add pasta to boiling water and cook according to package directions, until al dente (tender yet still firm to the bite).

4. Heat the remaining ¼ c. oil, anchovies and garlic in a 6-qt. pot or Dutch oven over medium-low heat. Cook 5 min., stirring until anchovies start to dissolve. Raise heat to medium; stir in wet escarole leaves in batches until incorporated. Cover pot; cook until escarole has wilted, about 3 min. Remove cover. Stir in beans, salt and pepper. Simmer mixture, stirring until most of the water has evaporated.

5. Drain pasta in colander; reserve 1 c. of the cooking water. Stir pasta into escarole mixture, moistening with some of the reserved cooking water as desired. Serve topped with toasted bread crumbs.

PER SERVING |||||||||||||||||||||||||||||||||||||||||||||||||||||||||||||||||||||||||||||||||||||||||||||||||||||||||||||

Calories 510 | Protein 17 g | Carbohydrate 77 g | Total fat 15 g

Sat fat 2 g | Fiber 14 g | Sodium 330 mg

Pizza Crust Panzanella

MAKES **4 SERVINGS**

1 (11- to 12-in.) thin 100% whole wheat pizza crust

2 pts. cherry tomatoes, cut in half

8 oz. fresh mini mozzarella balls, cut in quarters

¾ c. unsalted canned cannellini beans, drained

¼ c. thinly sliced packed fresh basil leaves

2 Tbsp. white wine vinegar

¼ tsp. salt

¼ tsp. pepper

1. Cut crust into 1-in. squares; in 12-in. skillet, cook on medium heat 10 min. or until browned and crisp, stirring occasionally. Cool.

2. In large bowl, combine cherry tomatoes, mozzarella, cannellini beans, basil, vinegar, and salt and pepper with crust pieces.

Dessert for One: 1 c. cantaloupe, cubed, served with 1 slice prosciutto.

PER SERVING ||||||||||||||||||||||||||||||||||||||||||||||||||||||||||||||||||||||||||||||||||||||||

Calories 480 | Protein 25 g | Carbohydrate 58 g | Total fat 19 g
Sat fat 10 g | Fiber 1 g | Sodium 940 mg

Quick Chicken Kebabs

MAKES **4 SERVINGS**

1 lb. boneless, skinless
  chicken thighs, cubed

3 Tbsp. olive oil

2 Tbsp. soy sauce

3 c. cubed pineapple

1 bunch green onions,
  cut into 1-in. pieces

¼ c. cider vinegar

1. Toss cubed chicken thighs, oil, and soy sauce; thread on soaked wooden skewers, alternating with cubed pineapple and green onions, and grill on medium-high, basting with cider vinegar, 10 min. or until chicken is cooked through (165°F), turning over once.

Side for One: ⅔ c. frozen brown rice, cooked; mixed with ⅓ red pepper, diced.

PER SERVING ||||||||||||||||||||||||||||||||||||||||||||||||||||||||||||||||||||||||||||||||||||||||

Calories 480 | Protein 25 g | Carbohydrate 48 g | Total fat 20 g
Sat fat 4 g | Fiber 4 g | Sodium 380 mg

Red Cabbage Spaghetti with Golden Raisins

MAKES **6 SERVINGS**

2½ tsp. Salt

1 head (about 1½ lbs.) red cabbage

1 Tbsp. olive oil

1 sm. onion, chopped

1 clove garlic, crushed with press

1 c. apple juice

½ c. golden raisins

Pinch ground cloves

8 oz. thin spaghetti

1. Heat large covered saucepot of cold water and 2 tsp. salt to boiling over high heat.

2. Meanwhile, discard any tough outer leaves from cabbage. Cut cabbage into quarters; cut core from each quarter. Thinly slice cabbage.

3. In nonstick 12-in. skillet, heat oil over medium heat. Add onion and cook about 8 min. or until tender, stirring occasionally. Add garlic and cook 1 min., stirring. Stir in cabbage, apple juice, raisins, cloves and ½ tsp. salt. Cover and cook about 15 min. or until cabbage is tender, stirring occasionally.

4. About 5 min. before cabbage is done, add pasta to boiling water and cook according to package directions.

5. Reserve ¼ c. pasta cooking water; drain pasta. Stir pasta into cabbage mixture in skillet; add cooking water if mixture seems dry.

Dessert for One: 20 grapes.

PER SERVING
Calories 510 | Protein 13 g | Carbohydrate 98 g | Total fat 11 g
Sat fat 1 g | Fiber 11 g | Sodium 55 mg

Rosemary-Rubbed Grilled Strip Steak with Blackberry Sauce

MAKES **6 SERVINGS**

3 Tbsp. olive oil

3 cloves garlic, crushed

1 tsp. dried rosemary

½ tsp. freshly ground black pepper

3 (1-in.-thick) boneless New York strip steaks (about 1½ lbs. total)

18 oz. blackberries, plus whole berries for garnish

3 Tbsp. Worcestershire sauce

3 Tbsp. balsamic vinegar

3 Tbsp. tomato paste

½ tsp. ground mustard

3 Tbsp. water

¼ tsp. salt, plus more to taste

⅛ tsp. cayenne pepper

2 (5-oz.) bags baby spinach

1. Prepare grill for direct grilling on medium-high.

2. Combine oil, garlic, rosemary and black pepper. Rub over steaks. Let stand 10 min.

3. Meanwhile, in a 2-qt. saucepan, combine blackberries, Worcestershire sauce, vinegar, tomato paste, mustard, water, salt and cayenne. Heat to simmering on medium. Simmer 5 to 7 min. or until berries have softened, stirring occasionally. With potato masher, carefully mash berries. Cool.

4. While sauce cools, sprinkle steaks with salt and grill 8 to 10 min. on medium (140°F), turning halfway through. Transfer to cutting board. Let stand 10 min.

5. Pour sauce through sieve set over medium bowl, pushing through with spoon. Discard solids. Thinly slice steak. Divide spinach among 6 plates and top with sliced steak. Serve with sauce. Garnish with whole berries.

Dessert for One: 1 Yasso Frozen Greek Yogurt popsicle (any 80-calorie variety).

PER SERVING ||||||||||||||||||||||||||||||||||||||||||||||||||||||||||||||||||||||||||||||||||||||||||||||||

Calories 480 | Protein 32 g | Carbohydrate 33 g | Total fat 25 g
Sat fat 8 g | Fiber 7 g | Sodium 340 mg

Shrimp Burgers with Mango-Avocado Salsa

MAKES **4 SERVINGS**

Mango-Avocado Salsa

1 sm. ripe mango,
    pitted, peeled and diced

1 sm. firm-ripe Hass
    avocado, pitted, peeled
    and diced

¼ c. red bell pepper

2 Tbsp. diced red onion

1½ Tbsp. fresh lime juice

1½ Tbsp. chopped cilantro

¼ tsp. kosher salt

¼ tsp. black pepper

Burgers

2 slices whole wheat
    bread, torn into pieces

1½ lbs. shrimp, chilled,
    peeled and deveined

2 Tbsp. coarsely chopped
    cilantro

2 Tbsp. snipped fresh chives

1 tsp. garlic paste, or half
    that amount pressed fresh
    garlic

¼ c. finely diced radish

¼ c. finely diced celery

2 Tbsp. low-fat mayonnaise

1 tsp. grated lemon zest

1 Tbsp. lemon juice

¾ tsp. kosher salt

¼ tsp. freshly ground black
    pepper

4 whole wheat sesame
    hamburger buns

1 c. mixed salad greens

1. *Salsa:* Combine all ingredients in a bowl.

2. *Burgers:* Pulse bread in a food processor until fine crumbs form; transfer to a bowl. Add shrimp, cilantro, chives and garlic paste to food processor and pulse until shrimp are finely chopped and form a chunky paste (do not puree—make sure to leave some texture).

3. Add shrimp mixture to bread crumbs along with radish, celery, mayo, lemon zest, lemon juice, salt and pepper; stir to combine. With moistened hands, gently shape 4 burgers, about 1 inch thick. Refrigerate burgers.

4. Prepare an outdoor grill with a medium-hot fire, or heat a stovetop grill pan over medium heat. Spray burgers on both sides with cooking spray. Grill 3 to 4 min. per side, until golden and just cooked through in centers. Toast buns on grill 1 to 2 min. Put salad greens on bun bottoms and top with burgers. Spoon salsa over burgers and cover with bun tops. Serve with remaining salsa.

PER SERVING

Calories 480 | Protein 41 g | Carbohydrate 47 g | Total fat 16 g
Sat fat 2 g | Fiber 8 g | Sodium 1,120 mg

Spicy Tuna Roll Salad

MAKES **4 MAIN DISH SERVINGS**

2 Tbsp. vegetable oil

1 (12-oz., about 1½-in.-thick) fresh tuna steak, or 2 (5- to 6-oz.) cans good-quality tuna in oil, drained

¼ tsp. salt

¼ tsp. pepper

¼ c. light mayonnaise

1 Tbsp. Asian hot chili sauce (such as sriracha)

1 Tbsp. fresh lime juice

1 Tbsp. soy sauce

1 Tbsp. toasted sesame oil

1 pinch sugar

6 c. arugula

2 c. cooked brown rice, cooled

1 seedless (English) cucumber, thinly sliced into half-moons

1 avocado, chopped

1. If using fresh tuna: In 10-in. skillet, heat vegetable oil on medium-high until very hot. Sprinkle tuna all over with salt and pepper. Add tuna to skillet; cook 3 min. per side or until browned on both sides. Transfer cooked tuna to cutting board. Thinly slice.

2. In large bowl, whisk together mayonnaise, chili sauce, lime juice, soy sauce, sesame oil and sugar. Add arugula, rice, cucumber and avocado; toss to combine. Divide salad among 4 serving plates. Top with tuna.

PER SERVING ||||||||||||||||||||||||||||||||||||||||||||||||||||||||||||||||||||||||||||||||||||||

Calories 490 | Protein 25 g | Carbohydrate 36 g | Total fat 28 g
Sat fat 4 g | Fiber 6 g | Sodium 800 mg

Sticky Glazed Salmon

MAKES **4 SERVINGS**

3 Tbsp. maple syrup

1 Tbsp. reduced-sodium soy sauce

2 tsp. rice wine vinegar

¼ tsp. ground ginger

4 (4-oz.) skinless salmon fillets

⅛ tsp. salt

¼ tsp. pepper

1. In small bowl, whisk together maple syrup, soy sauce, rice wine vinegar and ground ginger.

2. Sprinkle salmon fillets with salt and pepper.

3. Place salmon in 12-in. nonstick skillet; brush with some glaze. Cook on medium heat 9 to 10 min. or until just opaque throughout, generously brushing often with glaze and turning over once.

Side for One: ⅔ c. cooked quinoa mixed with 2 Tbsp. sliced almonds and 10 baby carrots, steamed and sprinkled with ½ tsp. reduced-sodium soy sauce.

PER SERVING

Calories 500 | Protein 32 g | Carbohydrate 48 g | Total fat 21 g
Sat fat 3 g | Fiber 8 g | Sodium 480 mg

Tuna Tomato Linguine

MAKES **4 SERVINGS**

1 lb. whole wheat linguine

1 lb. zucchini, trimmed

2 (5-oz.) cans tuna in olive oil, undrained

1 pt. cherry tomatoes, cut in half

2 Tbsp. capers, rinsed and chopped

¼ tsp. salt

¼ tsp. pepper

1. Cook linguine according to package directions. Meanwhile, with vegetable peeler, peel zucchini into wide ribbons. Drain pasta.

2. Toss pasta with zucchini, tuna and oil, tomatoes, capers, salt and pepper.

PER SERVING ||||||||||||||||||||||||||||||||||||||||||||||||||||||||||||||||||||||||||||||||||||||||||||||||||||||||||||||||||||

Calories 530 | Protein 40 g | Carbohydrate 92 g | Total fat 4 g Sat fat 0 g | Fiber 17 g | Sodium 620 mg

Turkey Vegetable Soup

MAKES **6 MAIN DISH SERVINGS**

1 Tbsp. olive oil

1 med. onion, chopped

3 med. carrots, cut into
½-in. chunks

2 med. stalks celery, cut
into ½-in. slices

1 c. frozen lima beans

6 c. chicken broth

¾ tsp. salt

¼ tsp. black pepper

2 c. cooked brown rice

1 ½ c. fresh corn kernels

2 c. (½-in. chunks) skinless
leftover cooked turkey

½ c. fresh parsley
leaves, chopped

1. In 4-qt. saucepan, heat oil. Add onion and cook 6 min. or until tender, stirring often.

2. Stir in carrots, celery, beans, broth, ¾ tsp. salt and ¼ tsp. ground black pepper; heat to boiling on high. Reduce heat to low and simmer 5 min. or until vegetables are tender.

3. Stir rice and corn into soup; heat to boiling. Stir in turkey and heat through. Remove saucepan from heat; stir in parsley.

Side for One: Mash ¼ avocado over 1 slice whole wheat bread; sprinkle with 1 Tbsp. grated Parmesan and heat in broiler until cheese melts.

PER SERVING |||||||||||||||||||||||||||||||||||||||||||||||||||||||||||||||||||||||||||||||||

Calories 500 | Protein 36 g | Carbohydrate 56 g | Total fat 15 g
Sat fat 2.5 g | Fiber 11 g | Sodium 1,310 mg

Turkey with Tomato & White Bean Ragu

MAKES **4 SERVINGS**

1 c. quinoa, rinsed and drained

3 Tbsp. sliced almonds

3 tsp. extra-virgin olive oil

1 lb. turkey breast cutlets

½ tsp. salt

½ tsp. pepper

1 sm. (4- to 6-oz.) onion, finely chopped

3 tsp. fresh oregano leaves, chopped, plus sprigs for garnish

2 pts. grape tomatoes, cut in half

1 clove garlic, crushed with press

1 (14- to 15-oz.) can no-salt-added white kidney beans, rinsed and drained

1. In 2-qt. saucepan, heat quinoa and 1½ c. water to boiling; reduce heat to medium. Cover; cook 15 min. or until liquid is absorbed. Stir in almonds.

2. Meanwhile, in 12-in. nonstick skillet, heat 2 tsp. oil on medium 1 min. Season turkey with ¼ tsp. each salt and freshly ground black pepper; add to skillet. Cook 7 min. or until browned on both sides, turning once. Transfer to plate.

3. To skillet, add onion, 2 tsp. oregano and remaining oil; cook 3 min., stirring. Stir in tomatoes and garlic; cook 5 min. or until softened. Stir in beans, ¼ tsp. salt and ¼ c. water. Cook 2 min. Add turkey; cook 3 min. or until no longer pink in center. Remove from heat; stir in remaining oregano.

4. Divide quinoa among serving plates; top with ragu and turkey. Garnish with oregano sprigs.

PER SERVING |||||||||||||||||||||||||||||||||||||||||||||||||||||||||||||||||||||||||||||||||||||||
Calories 520 | Protein 41 g | Carbohydrate 51 g | Total fat 17 g
Sat fat 2 g | Fiber 7 g | Sodium 290 mg

Tuscan Sun Salmon Salad

MAKES **4 SERVINGS**

1 lemon, thinly sliced

4 (5-oz.) skinless salmon fillets

¼ tsp. salt

⅛ tsp. freshly ground black pepper

5 oz. baby arugula

½ c. red peppers, sliced and roasted

½ c. Kalamata olives, pitted

1 Tbsp. balsamic vinegar

2 tsp. extra-virgin olive oil

1. Arrange, in 8" by 8" glass baking dish, thin slices of lemon in single layer.

2. Add ¼ c. water. Place salmon on top; sprinkle with salt and freshly ground black pepper.

3. Cover with vented plastic wrap and microwave on High 8 min. or until fish turns just opaque throughout. Meanwhile, in large bowl, toss baby arugula, roasted red peppers, Kalamata olives, balsamic vinegar and oil.

4. Divide salad among 4 plates and top with salmon.

Side for One: A small piece (1 oz.) focaccia.

PER SERVING |||||||||||||||||||||||||||||||||||||||||||||||||||||||||||||||||||||||||||||||||||||
Calories 470 | Protein 33 g | Carbohydrate 37 g | Total fat 21 g
Sat fat 3.5 g | Fiber 3 g | Sodium 720 mg

Vegetable Lasagna Toss

MAKES **4 SERVINGS**

8 oz. lasagna noodles

1 Tbsp. extra-virgin olive oil

2 cloves garlic, crushed
with press

1 (12-oz.) bag broccoli florets

1 c. low-sodium chicken
broth

1 (15- to 19-oz.) can white
kidney beans (cannel-
lini), drained and rinsed

3 large tomatoes, coarsely
chopped

⅓ c. freshly grated Romano
cheese, plus additional
for serving

1. Heat a 5- to 6-qt. covered saucepot of salted water to boiling over high heat. Add noodles and cook until just tender, about 2 min. longer than package directs.

2. Meanwhile, in nonstick 12-in. skillet, heat oil over medium heat; add garlic and broccoli, and cook 1 min., stirring frequently. Add broth; cover and cook 8 min. Stir in beans; cover and cook 2 to 3 min. longer or until broccoli is very tender. Stir in tomatoes; remove from heat.

3. Drain lasagna noodles; add to broccoli mixture in skillet and sprinkle with Romano. Toss to coat noodles. Serve with additional Romano if you like.

Side for One: Salad made with 2 c. mixed greens, 5 cherry tomatoes, ¼ cucumber, sliced; top with 1 Tbsp. grated Parmesan and 1 Tbsp. light balsamic vinaigrette.

PER SERVING ||||||||||||||||||||||||||||||||||||||||||||||||||||||||||||||||||||||||||||||||||||||||||

Calories 500 | Protein 24 g | Carbohydrate 75 g | Total fat 12 g
Sat fat 3.5 g | Fiber 20 g | Sodium 550 mg

Snacks

Creating a 100- or 200-calorie snack is easy—just go to this list. It offers plenty of variety, and there are two weeks' worth of suggestions for each calorie range. Stick with the 100-calorie snacks if your allotment of calories per day is only 1,400. If your allowance is higher, you can choose more than one 100-calorie snack or a 200-calorie snack. Remember to keep track of all of the calories you consume —including wine if you choose it in lieu of a snack—in order to stay within your daily calorie allowance. The best time for a snack is between lunch and dinner, when you typically go the longest between meals, but try to have it before 3 P.M.

100 calories

Asian app » ½ c. edamame

Chocolaty-orange fix » 1 orange served with 5 Blue Diamond oven-roasted dark-chocolate almonds

Diner-style nosh » 1 VitaMuffin muffin top (any variety)

Frozen treat: Yasso Greek yogurt bar (any flavor)

Frozen yogurt » Freeze 1 Chobani Bite cup (any variety) for 30 min. before eating

Hors d'oeuvres for one » ¼ cucumber, sliced, spread with 1½ Tbsp. goat cheese and topped with 1 oz. lox divided among slices

Hummus with dippers » 2 Tbsp. hummus served with ½ red pepper, sliced

Mediterranean meze » BelGioioso Fresh Mozzarella Snacking Cheese with 5 cherry tomatoes

Mexi snack » 2 Tbsp. guacamole served with 10 baby carrots

Movie treat » 2½ c. SmartPop! popcorn or 3¼ c. air-popped popcorn

NY special » ½ bagel thin (such as Thomas') spread with 1 Laughing Cow Light cheese wedge (any variety)

Pear "fondue" » 1½ tsp. hazelnut butter spread among the bottom halves of slices from ½ pear

Protein picker-upper » 1 hard-boiled egg seasoned with 1 tsp. sriracha and served with ½ c. low-sodium vegetable juice

Or, if you choose an alcoholic beverage » 5 oz. wine, 1½ oz. spirit or 12 oz. beer (around 125 calories)

200 calories

Banana split » Split a banana lengthwise; spread one side with 1 tsp. hazelnut spread and the other side with 1 tsp. peanut butter. Top with 1 whole-grain graham cracker square, crumbled.

Power bar » 1 KIND Dark Chocolate Nuts & Sea Salt bar or Über Dark Chocolate Peanut bar

Cheese and crackers » 1 reduced-fat cheese stick served with 6 Triscuits

Chips and dip » 1 Tbsp. guacamole served with 8 whole-grain corn tortilla chips

Chocolaty waffle » Top a toasted whole-grain waffle with 1 Tbsp. hazelnut butter and ¼ c. strawberries, sliced

Coffee-shop stop » 1 16-oz. skim latte and ½ banana

Ice cream sundae » ½ c. Edy's Slow-Churned Classic Vanilla ice cream topped with ¼ c. strawberries, sliced, and 1½ Tbsp. dry roasted peanuts

Mediterranean melon bowl »2 c. watermelon, cubed, mixed with ¼ c. feta crumbles

Munchie madness »18 SunChips served with ¼ c. Oikos French Onion Dip

Peach pie »Top a sliced peach with ¼ c. plain nonfat Greek yogurt, 1 tsp. honey and 1 crushed whole-grain graham cracker rectangle

Piña colada smoothie »In blender, whirl 1 c. frozen pineapple with ¼ c. plain nonfat Greek yogurt, ½ c. fat-free milk, 1 tsp. honey and 2 tsp. shredded, unsweetened coconut

Sampler plate »1 c. cherries served with ¾ oz. Brie and 2 Triscuits

Sweet and salty »1 apple spread with 1 Tbsp. nut butter

Trail mix »¼ c. walnut halves and 1½ Tbsp. golden raisins

chapter 10 Sides and Desserts

ON THE GIRLFRIENDS DIET, there is the option of adding sides and/or dessert to your meals. We've suggested some possible sides and desserts in the meal plan and this chapter includes those recipes along with other options. Some of these recipes have substantial numbers of calories, so reserve them for special occasions. While you are on the meal plan, keep in mind that it allows you 500 calories each for lunch and dinner; if your burn rate allows you to consume more calories, use some of these recipes to supplement the basic meal plan. Just remember not to exceed your total daily calorie consumption represented by your personal RMR that you figured out from the formulas in Chapter 2, minus the number of calories you are cutting back to achieve your weight loss goal.

Broccoli-Cauliflower Roast

MAKES **6 SERVINGS**

2 med. (1½-lb.) heads broccoli, cut into florets

2½ Tbsp. extra-virgin olive oil

½ tsp. salt, plus more to taste

¼ tsp. freshly ground black pepper, plus more to taste

1 sm. (1¼-lb.) head cauliflower, cut into florets

1 sm. orange

1 sm. lemon

⅛ c. pitted green olives, thinly sliced

1 Tbsp. fresh flat-leaf parsley leaves, chopped, for garnish

1. Arrange 2 oven racks in bottom half of oven. Preheat oven to 450°F.

2. On 18" by 12" baking pan, toss broccoli with 1 Tbsp. oil, ¼ tsp. salt and ⅛ tsp. pepper. On another 18" by 12" baking pan, toss cauliflower with 1 Tbsp. oil, ¼ tsp. salt, and ⅛ tsp. pepper.

3. Roast 30 to 35 min. or until vegetables are browned and just tender, rotating pans between racks halfway through roasting.

4. Meanwhile, from orange, grate ½ tsp. peel and squeeze ¼ c. juice into medium bowl. Into same bowl, from lemon, grate ¼ tsp. peel and squeeze 2 Tbsp. juice. Whisk in remaining oil, salt to taste and add a pinch of pepper.

5. Arrange broccoli and cauliflower on serving platter. Scatter olives over vegetables. Whisk dressing again and drizzle all over dish. Garnish with parsley.

PER SERVING ||||||||||||||||||||||||||||||||||||||||||||||||||||||||||||||||||||||||||||||||||||||||
Calories 160 | Protein 9 g | Carbohydrate 21 g | Total fat 8 g
Sat fat 1 g | Fiber 10 g | Sodium 380 mg

Brussels Sprouts with Shallots

MAKES **6 SERVINGS**

1¼ lbs. brussels sprouts, trimmed and halved

1 Tbsp. olive oil

2 shallots, diced

¼ tsp. salt, plus more to taste

1 tsp. sugar

2 Tbsp. white wine vinegar

½ c. low-sodium chicken broth

⅛ tsp. freshly ground black pepper

1 Tbsp. snipped chives

1. Fill large covered saucepot with salted water and bring to a boil on high heat. Fill large bowl with ice and water. Add brussels sprouts to pot. Cook 5 min. or until bright green and just tender. (A knife should pierce through core with little resistance.) Drain; transfer to ice water. When cool, drain again (brussels sprouts can be covered and refrigerated up to 2 days).

2. In same large pot, on medium heat, add half the oil. Add shallots and a few sprinkles salt, and cook 2 to 5 min. or until tender, stirring frequently.

3. Add sugar and vinegar, and stir well. Cook until liquid evaporates. Stir in broth, increase heat to high, and boil until mixture is almost dry.

4. Reduce heat to medium. Stir in remaining oil, salt and pepper. Return drained brussels sprouts to pot. Cook until heated through, stirring frequently. Transfer to serving dish and top with chives.

PER SERVING ||||||||||||||||||||||||||||||||||||||||||||||||||||||||||||||||||||||||||||||||||

Calories 70 | Protein 4 g | Carbohydrate 10 g | Total fat 2.5 g
Sat fat 0 g | Fiber 4 g | Sodium 30 mg

Butternut Squash Fries

MAKES **4 SERVINGS**

1 (2-lb.) butternut squash
½ tsp. sea salt
½ tsp. cinnamon

1. Preheat oven to 425°F. Meanwhile, cut both ends off squash and discard. Cut in half and remove seeds. Peel with vegetable peeler. Using a crinkle cutter or knife, cut squash into spears the size of steak fries. Pat dry with a paper towel. Lay spears on a dry paper towel and sprinkle with salt. Let stand 5 min. Blot with dry paper towel.

2. Spray baking sheet with nonstick spray. Place spears on sheet and sprinkle with cinnamon. Bake for 20 min. Remove fries from oven, flip with a spatula, and return to oven and cook 20 min. more, or until crispy on the outside.

PER SERVING ||||||||||||||||||||||||||||||||||||||||||||||||||||||||||||||||||||||||||||||||||||||
Calories 100 | Protein 2 g | Carbohydrate 27 g | Total fat 0 g
Sat fat 0 g | Fiber 5 g | Sodium 300 mg

Chunky Vegetable Bulgur Salad

MAKES **8 SERVINGS**

2 c. bulgur

2½ c. boiling water

2 lemons

1 Tbsp. olive oil

1 sm. red onion, finely chopped

1 c. cherry tomatoes, halved

1 med. (8-oz.) zucchini, chopped

1 med. (8-oz.) yellow summer squash, chopped

½ c. (loosely packed) fresh mint leaves, chopped

½ c. (loosely packed) fresh parsley leaves, chopped

½ tsp. salt

¼ tsp. coarsely ground black pepper

1. In large bowl, stir together bulgur and boiling water. Cover and let stand 30 min. or until liquid is absorbed.

2. Meanwhile, from lemons, grate 1 tsp. peel and squeeze ¼ c. juice; set aside. In nonstick 12-in. skillet, heat oil over medium-high heat until hot. Add onion and cook 3 to 4 min. or until beginning to soften. Add tomatoes, zucchini and squash, and cook 6 to 8 min. or until vegetables are tender, stirring occasionally.

3. Stir vegetables into bulgur with lemon peel and juice, mint, parsley, salt and pepper. Spoon into container with tight-fitting lid. Can be refrigerated up to 1 day.

PER SERVING ||||||||||||||||||||||||||||||||||||||||||||||||||||||||||||||||||||||||||||||||||||||||||

Calories 160 | Protein 6 g | Carbohydrate 32 g | Total fat 2.5 g
Sat fat 0 g | Fiber 8 g | Sodium 90 mg

Creamy Cole Slaw

MAKES **4 SERVINGS**

1 (16-oz.) bag cole slaw mix

¼ c. fat-free mayonnaise

¼ c. fat-free sour cream

2½ Tbsp. seasoned rice vinegar

1 Tbsp. granulated sugar

1 tsp. Dijonnaise

¼ tsp. seasoned salt

1. Combine all ingredients in large bowl. Cover and chill in refrigerator for at least 3 hours.

PER SERVING ||||||||||||||||||||||||||||||||||||||||||||||||||||||||||||||||||||||||||||||||
Calories 70 | Protein 2 g | Carbohydrate 16 g | Total fat 0.5 g
Sat fat 0 g | Fiber 3 g | Sodium 510 mg

Grilled Melon Salad

MAKES **4 SERVINGS**

3 c. melon chunks

3 Tbsp. olive oil

Salt and pepper to taste

4 c. arugula

3 slices cooked crispy extra-lean bacon, crumbled

½ c. fresh basil leaves

1. Prepare grill for direct grilling on medium-high. Thread melon chunks onto skewers. Brush with 1 Tbsp. oil, and sprinkle with salt and pepper. Grill 3 minutes, turning over once.

2. Toss greens with remaining oil. Place a skewer on top. Sprinkle with bacon and basil.

PER SERVING ||||||||||||||||||||||||||||||||||||||||||||||||||||||||||||||||||||||||||||||||
Calories 190 | Protein 6 g | Carbohydrate 14 g | Total fat 12 g
Sat fat 2 g | Fiber 2 g | Sodium 430 mg

Kale Ribbons with Dates & Olives

MAKES **4 SERVINGS**

1 bunch kale

½ c. pitted dates, cut into slivers

⅓ c. toasted sliced almonds

¼ c. pitted green olives, sliced

2 Tbsp. extra-virgin olive oil

2 Tbsp. fresh lemon juice

⅛ tsp. salt

1. Remove and discard kale stems and thick ribs. Stack leaves, roll tightly and slice into ribbons. Put in salad bowl with dates, almonds and olives.

2. Whisk together olive oil, lemon juice and salt. Pour over salad and toss.

PER SERVING ||||||||||||||||||||||||||||||||||||||||||||||||||||||||||||||||||||||||||||||||||||||||||
Calories 210 | Protein 4 g | Carbohydrate 26 g | Total fat 13 g
Sat fat 1.5 g | Fiber 4 g | Sodium 240 mg

Red Potatoes over Greens

MAKES **8 SERVINGS**

1 lb. red potatoes, unpeeled and cut into ¼-in.-thick slices

1 c. sun-dried tomatoes (not packed in oil), cut in half

¼ c. extra-virgin olive oil

2½ Tbsp. lemon juice

1 lg. clove garlic, finely minced

1 Tbsp. chopped fresh oregano

Salt and pepper to taste

1 c. sliced seedless cucumber

½ c. sliced red onion

1 c. crumbled feta cheese

½ c. pitted Greek olives

6 c. mixed greens

1. In large pot of water, bring potatoes to a boil; reduce heat and simmer until potatoes are tender; drain.

2. Pour boiling water over sun-dried tomatoes in bowl; set aside. In large bowl, whisk olive oil, ¼ c. water, lemon juice, garlic, oregano, salt and pepper.

3. Drain tomatoes and pat dry. Toss potatoes, tomatoes and cucumber with dressing. Add onion, feta and olives, and toss. Refrigerate until serving time. Plate greens, and top with potato salad.

PER SERVING ||||||||||||||||||||||||||||||||||||||||||||||||||||||||||||||||||||||||||||||||||||||||
Calories 200 | Protein 6 g | Carbohydrate 18 g | Total fat 12 g
Sat fat 4 g | Fiber 3 g | Sodium 320 mg

Roasted Beet & Olive Salad with Orange & Mint

MAKES **10 SERVINGS**

6 med. (2 lbs. total) beets (red and golden), without tops, rinsed

3 Tbsp. extra-virgin olive oil

3 Tbsp. white balsamic vinegar

2 cloves garlic, crushed through a press

1 tsp. kosher salt

½ tsp. freshly ground black pepper

¼ tsp. ground allspice

1 c. oil-cured black olives

1 navel orange, thinly sliced, slices cut into small triangles

2 Tbsp. fresh mint leaves

1. Heat oven to 400°F. Wrap red and golden beets separately in foil packets. Roast 1 hr. or until tender. Cool to room temperature. Peel beets; cut into ¾-in. dice.

2. In large serving bowl, whisk oil, vinegar, garlic, salt, pepper and allspice; add beets, olives and orange triangles. Gently toss.

3. Let marinate at room temperature for 1 hr. before serving. Stir in mint before serving.

PER SERVING ||||||||||||||||||||||||||||||||||||||||||||||||||||||||||||||||||||||||||||||||||||||||||||

Calories 100 | Protein 2 g | Carbohydrate 12 g | Total fat 6 g
Sat fat 1 g | Fiber 3 g | Sodium 380 mg

Roasted Vegetables

Appreciating vegetables is at the core of the Mediterranean diet. We've found that a great way to get the most flavor and, in our humble view, the most satisfaction out of vegetables is by roasting them. When vegetables meet the high, dry heat of the oven, their natural sugars caramelize, transforming them into richly satisfying dishes. For every 2 lbs. vegetables, toss with 1 Tbsp. olive oil prior to roasting, and add salt and freshly ground black pepper to taste. Spread in a single layer with space between. Roasted vegetables are a perfect accompaniment to chicken, beef and pork. Two pounds of vegetables is six servings.

VEGETABLE	HOW TO CUT	ROASTING TIME AT 450°F	SEASONING	CALORIES PER SERVING
ASPARAGUS	In 1-inch-long pieces	10 to 15 minutes	Sprinkle with 1 tsp. freshly grated lemon peel after roasting.	51
BEETS	Use small beets and roast them whole	30 to 40 minutes	Peel beets and sprinkle with 1 Tbsp. chopped fresh basil and 1 Tbsp. balsamic vinegar after roasting.	67
BELL PEPPERS	In 1-inch-wide strips	30 minutes	Sprinkle with 3 large fresh basil leaves, thinly sliced, after roasting.	68
BROCCOLI	Trim and peel stem; split florets into 1½- to 2-inch-wide pieces.	10 to 15 minutes	Sprinkle with 1 Tbsp. grated Cheddar cheese after roasting.	63
CARROTS	In In ½-inch-thick slices	20 to 25 minutes	Drizzle with 1 Tbsp. orange juice after roasting.	63

VEGETABLE	HOW TO CUT	ROASTING TIME AT 450°F	SEASONING	CALORIES PER SERVING
EGGPLANT	In ½-inch-thick slices	20 to 25 minutes	Drizzle with 1 Tbsp. extra virgin olive oil after roasting.	57
FENNEL	Trimmed and cut into wedges	35 to 40 minutes	Sprinkle with ½ tsp. freshly grated orange peel after roasting.	68
GREEN BEANS	Trimmed	20 to 30 minutes	Toss with 2 Tbsp. each fresh lemon juice and chopped fresh dill after roasting.	68
ONIONS	Each cut into 12 wedges	20 to 30 minutes	Brush with mixture of 1 Tbsp. brown sugar, 1 tsp. cider vinegar; roast 5 minutes more.	67
PARSNIPS	Each cut into ½-inch pieces	30 minutes	Drizzle with 1 Tbsp. balsamic vinegar	115
POTATOES	In 2-inch pieces	45 minutes	Sprinkle with ½ tsp. freshly grated orange peel after roasting.	133
SWEET POTATOES	Cut crosswise in half, then lengthwise into 1-inch wedges	30 minutes	Toss with 2 Tbsp. chopped fresh rosemary before roasting.	151
ZUCCHINI	Trimmed and cut in half crosswise, then each half quartered	15 to 20 minutes	Top with 1 Tbsp. freshly grated Parmesan cheese.	45

Spinach Sauté

MAKES **8 SERVINGS**

1 Tbsp. olive oil

2 cloves garlic, crushed

2 (10-oz.) bags spinach, rinsed but not dried

1 Tbsp. fresh lemon juice

¼ tsp. salt

1. Heat oil in 6-qt. saucepot on medium-high until hot. Add garlic and cook 1 min., or until golden, stirring. Add spinach in batches. Cook 2 min. or until all spinach fits in saucepot. Cover and cook 2 to 3 min. longer, or just until spinach wilts, stirring once. Remove from heat. Stir in lemon juice and salt.

PER SERVING |||||||||||||||||||||||||||||||||||||||||||||||||||||||||||||||||||||||||||||||
Calories 45 | Protein 2 g | Carbohydrate 8 g | Total fat 2 g
Sat fat 0 g | Fiber 3 g | Sodium 190 mg

Tropical Fruit Salad

MAKES **6 SERVINGS**

⅓ c. fresh lime juice

1½ Tbsp. honey

¾ tsp. chopped fresh ginger

1 c. blueberries

1 c. bananas, sliced

1 c. pineapple chunks

1 c. cubed mango

1 c. raspberries

1 c. blackberries

1. In large bowl, stir together lime juice, honey and ginger. Add fruit and toss. If using bananas, serve immediately.

PER SERVING |||||||||||||||||||||||||||||||||||||||||||||||||||||||||||||||||||||||||||||||
Calories 100 | Protein 1 g | Carbohydrate 27 g | Total fat 0.5 g
Sat fat 0 g | Fiber 5 g | Sodium 0 mg

Desserts

Dessert doesn't have to be a diet buster. When visions of sweet some-things pop in your head and won't move out, give in to one of these healthy and dessert-satisfying choices.

APPLE CRISP

Place 1 c. coarsely chopped Granny Smith apple and 2 tsp. apricot all-fruit preserves in 8-oz. teacup and microwave at 50% power for 3 min., stirring every 30 sec.; top with 2 Tbsp. low-fat granola and 1 Tbsp. nonfat vanilla Greek yogurt. PER SERVING | Calories 150 | Protein 3 g Carbohydrate 36 g | Total fat 1 g | Sat fat 0 g | Fiber 4 g | Sodium 40 mg

POMEGRANATE POACHED PEARS SIMMER

1 cinnamon stick, 4 c. pomegranate juice, 6 peeled, halved and cored pears and ¼ c. sugar in 4-qt. saucepan for 15 to 25 min. Serve with a dollop sour cream and a sprig of mint. Serves 6. PER SERVING | Calories 230 Protein 2 g | Carbohydrate 57 g | Total fat 1 g | Sat fat 0 g | Fiber 6 g | Sodium 25 mg

Fruit Swaps

Next to the taste, what we love best about fruit is the wide variety that can be eaten for 100 calories or less. Substitute any of these as a snack or dessert:

50 calories	100 calories
✳ 1 cup blueberries	✳ 1 medium apple
✳ 1 cup cantaloupe	✳ 1 medium banana
✳ ½ grapefruit	✳ 1 cup cherries
✳ 1 cup honeydew chunks	✳ 1 cup grapes
✳ 1 kiwifruit	✳ 1 small pear
✳ 1 small orange	
✳ 1 cup raspberries	
✳ 15 strawberries	

Brandy-Poached Winter Fruit with Cinnamon & Star Anise

MAKES **18 SERVINGS**

1 to 2 lg. navel oranges

½ c. sugar

½ c. brandy (optional)

1 cinnamon stick

1 whole star anise

2 lg. ripe Bartlett pears

1 lg. Granny Smith apple

1 lg. Gala or Fuji apple

1 c. dried Calimyrna figs, cut in quarters

1 c. dried apricots, halved

1 c. dried plums (prunes)

¼ c. dried sour cherries

1. With vegetable peeler, from orange(s), remove 3 strips peel (each 3 in. long) and squeeze ¾ c. juice. Set orange peels and juice aside separately.

2. In 4-qt. saucepan, combine 3½ c. water, sugar, brandy, cinnamon, star anise and reserved orange peel. Cover and heat to boiling on high; reduce heat to medium and simmer 5 min.

3. Meanwhile, peel and core pears and apples, then cut each fruit into ¼-in.-thick slices.

4. Stir figs, apricots, plums and cherries into saucepan; simmer 5 min. Stir in pears and apples; simmer 10 min. or until fruit is tender but not mushy, stirring occasionally.

5. Remove compote from heat and stir in reserved orange juice. Let stand at least 30 min. or up to 2 hr. Discard orange peel, star anise and cinnamon before serving.

PER SERVING ||||||||||||||||||||||||||||||||||||||||||||||||||||||||||||||||||||||||||||||||||||||||
Calories 130 | Protein 1 g | Carbohydrate 29 g | Total fat 0 g
Sat fat 0 g | Fiber 4 g | Sodium 0 mg

Buttermilk Panna Cotta with Blackberry Sauce

MAKES **8 SERVINGS**

1 envelope unflavored gelatin

2¾ c. buttermilk

½ c. plus 4 tsp. sugar

1 (10-oz.) bag frozen
  blackberries, thawed

1 tsp. fresh lemon juice

1. In cup, evenly sprinkle gelatin over ¼ c. water. Let stand 2 min. to allow gelatin to absorb liquid and soften.

2. In 3-qt. saucepan, heat ½ c. buttermilk and ½ c. sugar on medium 2 to 3 min. or until sugar dissolves, stirring occasionally. Reduce heat to low; whisk in gelatin. Cook 1 to 2 min., or until gelatin dissolves, stirring. Remove saucepan from heat; stir in remaining buttermilk.

3. Pour buttermilk mixture into eight 4-oz. ramekins. Place ramekins on rimmed baking pan. Cover pan with plastic wrap and refrigerate at least 4 hours or overnight, until well chilled and set.

4. Reserve ⅓ c. blackberries for garnish. In blender, puree remaining blackberries with lemon juice, 2 Tbsp. water and remaining sugar. Pour puree through sieve set over bowl, stirring to press out fruit sauce; discard seeds. Cover and refrigerate if not serving right away.

5. To unmold panna cotta, run tip of knife around edge of each ramekin. With hand, sharply tap side of each ramekin to break seal; invert onto 8 dessert plates. Spoon sauce around each panna cotta. Garnish with reserved berries.

PER SERVING ||||||||||||||||||||||||||||||||||||||||||||||||||||||||||||||||||||||||||
Calories 110 | Protein 5 g | Carbohydrate 21 g | Total fat 2 g
Sat fat 1 g | Fiber 2 g | Sodium 70 mg

Chocolate Pudding Cake

MAKES **5 SERVINGS**

1 (15-count) box
of frozen phyllo shells

1 (60-calorie) prepared
pudding snack

1. Prepare phyllo according to package directions.

2. Spoon an equal amount of pudding into each shell. If not eating immediately, refrigerate for up to 2 days.

PER SERVING ||||||||||||||||||||||||||||||||||||||||||||||||||||||||||||||||||||||||||||||||||||||||||||
Calories 70 | Protein 1 g | Carbohydrate 12 g | Total fat 2 g
Sat fat 0 g | Fiber 0 g | Sodium 125 mg

Greek Yogurt Four Ways

Easy add-ins transform a plain 6-oz. serving into a luscious, creamy treat fit for dessert or breakfast. It's fun, fast and easy:

BLUEBERRY & GRAHAM CRACKER Stir into yogurt ¼ c. each blueberries and cinnamon-flavored graham crackers, crushed, 1 Tbsp. honey and ¼ tsp. vanilla extract. Per serving: Calories 260, Protein 17 g, Carbohydrate 45 g, Total fat 2.5 g Sat fat 0 g, Fiber 2 g, Sodium 190 mg

CHOCOLATE & RASPBERRY Stir in 2 Tbsp. chocolate-hazelnut spread and 1 tsp. raspberry jam; garnish with fresh raspberries. Per serving: Calories 310, Protein 17 g Carbohydrate 35 g, Total fat 11 g, Sat fat 11 g, Fiber 3 g, Sodium 80 mg

PEACH & TOASTED ALMOND Microwave 2 Tbsp. sliced almonds on plate 1 min. or until toasted. Mix 1 sliced peach and 1 Tbsp. brown sugar in bowl; spoon over yogurt. Top with almonds. Per serving: Calories 270, Protein 18 g, Carbohydrate 38 g, Total fat 6 g, Sat fat 0 g, Fiber 3 g, Sodium 70 mg

PIÑA COLADA Microwave ¼ c. sweetened shredded coconut on High on plate, 1 to 2 min., until toasted; spoon over yogurt with ½ c. chopped pineapple. Per serving: Calories 250, Protein 16 g, Carbohydrate 29 g, Total fat 8 g, Sat fat 7 g, Fiber 2 g, Sodium 125 mg

Fire-Roasted Nectarines with Berry Salsa

MAKES **4 SERVINGS**

2 c. strawberries, hulled
and coarsely chopped

½ c. raspberries

⅓ c. blueberries

2 Tbsp. sugar

2 tsp. finely chopped
crystallized ginger

1 tsp. fresh lemon juice

Salt

4 ripe med. nectarines,
each cut in half and
pitted

1. Prepare berry salsa: In medium bowl, mix strawberries, raspberries, blueberries, sugar, ginger, lemon juice and pinch salt. Set aside.

2. Preheat outdoor grill to medium (or use indoor grill pan). Spray cut sides of nectarine halves with olive oil cooking spray. Place nectarine halves on hot grill and cook 5 to 6 min., or until fruit is lightly charred and tender, turning once.

3. To serve, in each of 4 dessert bowls, place 2 nectarine halves, cut sides up, and top with berry salsa.

PER SERVING |||||||||||||||||||||||||||||||||||||||||||||||||||||||||||||||||||||||||||||||||||||||
Calories 120 | Protein 2 g | Carbohydrate 31 g | Total fat 1 g
Sat fat 0 g | Fiber 6 g | Sodium 0 mg

Pears Baked in Red Wine

MAKES **6 SERVINGS**

1 lg. (12- to 14-oz.)
navel orange

6 (8-oz.) Bosc pears

½ c. hearty red wine
(such as Chianti)

¼ c. sugar

1 Tbsp. margarine,
melted

1. Preheat oven to 450°F. With vegetable peeler, remove peel from orange in 2" by 1½"strips.

2. With melon baller or small knife, remove cores and seeds from pears by cutting through blossom end (bottom) of unpeeled pears (do not remove stems from pears).

3. In shallow 1½- to 2-qt. glass or ceramic baking dish, combine orange peel, wine and ¼ c. water. Place sugar in medium bowl. Hold pears, one at a time, over bowl of sugar with one hand (keep other hand dry). With dry hand, use pastry brush to coat pears with melted margarine, then sprinkle pears with sugar until coated. Stand pears in baking dish. Sprinkle any remaining sugar into baking dish around pears.

4. Bake pears 35 to 40 min. or until tender when pierced with tip of a small knife, basting occasionally with syrup in baking dish.

5. Cool pears slightly, about 30 min., to serve warm. Or cool completely; refrigerate up to 1 day. Reheat to serve warm, if you like.

PER SERVING |||||||||||||||||||||||||||||||||||||||||||||||||||||||||||||||||||||||||||||||
Calories 220 | Protein 1 g | Carbohydrate 50 g | Total fat 2 g
Sat fat 0 g | Fiber 8 g | Sodium 20 mg

Better for You Ice Cream

We turned our office into a mini scoop shop to test the best guilt-free treats for you.
Yes, that's how much we care.

Ben & Jerry's Banana Peanut Butter Greek Frozen Yogurt

Serving size: ½ cup

Calories: 210

If you're looking for something truly light, Ben and Jerry aren't your dudes. But at least you get healthy bacteria and protein in their Greek yogurt varieties. And wow, are they good: "Like Pinkberry fro-yo on crack," said one tester. "Tart, sweet and creamy."

Blue Bunny Mini Swirls Chocolate Ice Cream Cones

Serving size: 1 cone

Calories: 140

Like the ice cream cones you remember having as a kid, but smaller and easier on the waistline. One GF said it best: "Hooray for snack size! Just the right portion."

Cadbury Caramello Ice Cream Bars

Serving size: 1 bar

Calories: 160

If you want something decadent, this mini bar is the way to go. Despite the reasonable size and calorie count, one tester thought it was "so yummy and rich, I couldn't finish it!"

✻ Order a copy of *The Girlfriends Diet* for your friend at goodhousekeeping.com/girlfriends.

✻ Share your success stories and get more dieting tips on our Facebook page at facebook.com/girlfriendsdiet.

chapter 11 Appetizers and Beverages

THERE'S SOMETHING FUN about skipping dinner and grazing on appetizers when you get together for a Girls' Night In. Here are half a dozen ideas to choose from, ranging in calories from 25 to 180. As you plan your evening—whether with your Girlfriends Diet Club or another social occasion—remember to keep tabs on the total number of calories of all the available food and drinks. One strategy is to think of the appetizers as replacing your dinnertime calories, so shoot for about 500 calories a person. If you are having 10 people over, you might want to choose appetizers that add up to 400 calories per person since that allows for everyone to have a glass of wine as well. But if you decide to make the sangria at 170 calories a serving, for example, you'll need to lower the quantity of appetizers you offer.

Artichoke & Mint Dip

YIELD **3 CUPS** | SERVING SIZE **1 TABLESPOON**

1 lemon

2 (13.75- to 14-oz.) cans artichoke hearts, drained

½ c. freshly grated Pecorino
Romano cheese

½ c. nonfat plain Greek
yogurt

¼ c. (loosely packed) fresh
mint leaves, plus additional
chopped mint for garnish

3 Tbsp. olive oil

Toasted baguette slices,
grape tomatoes, and yel-
low peppers, for serving

1. From lemon, grate 1 tsp. zest and squeeze
1 Tbsp. juice.

2. In food processor with knife blade attached,
blend lemon peel and juice, artichoke hearts,
Pecorino Romano, Greek yogurt, mint and oil
until smooth. If not serving right away, refrigerate up to 3 days.

3. To serve, spoon dip into serving bowl; garnish
with chopped mint. Serve with toast and vegetables.

PER SERVING |||||||||||||||||||||||||||||||||||||||||||||||||||||||||||||||||||||||||||||||||||||
Calories 25 | Protein 1 g | Carbohydrate 1 g | Total fat 2 g
Sat fat 1 g | Fiber 0 g | Sodium 55 mg

Fast-Fix Pea Dip

MAKES **12 SERVINGS**

1 Tbsp. olive oil

2 med. shallots, chopped

1 clove garlic, peeled

¼ tsp. plus ⅛ tsp. salt

10 oz. frozen peas

½ c. light sour cream

¼ c. fresh flat-leaf parsley
leaves

3 Tbsp. roasted, salted
almonds, plus more
for garnish

3 Tbsp. nonfat plain
Greek yogurt

1 Tbsp. fresh lemon juice

1 Tbsp. fresh tarragon
leaves, plus chopped
tarragon for garnish

⅛ tsp. freshly ground black
pepper

Assorted spring vegetables,
such as baby carrots,
sugar snap peas and
asparagus, for dipping

1. In 12-in. skillet, heat oil on medium. Add shallots, garlic, 2 Tbsp. water, and ⅛ tsp. salt. Cover and cook 4 to 6 min. or until very soft and browned, stirring occasionally. Stir in peas. Remove from heat; cool completely.

2. In food processor, pulse cooled shallot mixture, sour cream, parsley, almonds, Greek yogurt, lemon juice, tarragon, remaining salt and pepper until smooth.

3. Transfer to serving bowl. Cover with plastic wrap and refrigerate at least 1 hr. (or until cold) or up to 1 day. Garnish with almonds and chopped tarragon. Serve with spring vegetables.

PER SERVING ||||||||||||||||||||||||||||||||||||||||||||||||||||||||||||||||||||||||

Calories 85 | Protein 2 g | Carbohydrate 5 g | Total fat 6 g
Sat fat 1 g | Fiber 1 g | Sodium 135 mg

Goat Cheese & Tomato Bruschetta

MAKES **18 SERVINGS**

1 (8-oz.) loaf whole wheat baguette

1 (5½-oz.) pkg. soft mild goat cheese (such as Montrachet)

1 tsp. fresh oregano leaves, minced

¼ tsp. coarsely ground black pepper

2 med. ripe tomatoes, seeded and diced

⅛ tsp. salt

3 Tbsp. olive oil

2 tsp. fresh parsley leaves, minced

2 cloves garlic, each cut in half

1. Prepare charcoal fire or preheat gas grill for direct grilling over medium heat. Cut off ends from loaf of bread; reserve for making bread crumbs another day. Slice loaf diagonally into ½-in.-thick slices.

2. In small bowl, with fork, stir goat cheese, oregano and pepper until blended. In medium bowl, stir tomatoes with salt, 1 tsp. olive oil and 1 tsp. parsley.

3. Place bread slices on grill rack and cook 2 to 3 min. on each side, until lightly toasted. Rub 1 side of each toast slice with cut side of garlic. Brush with remaining olive oil.

4. Just before serving, spread goat-cheese mixture on toast and top with tomato mixture. Sprinkle with remaining parsley.

PER SERVING ||||||||||||||||||||||||||||||||||||||||||||||||||||||||||||||||||||||||||||||||||||||||||
Calories 180 | Protein 6 g | Carbohydrate 16 g | Total fat 10 g
Sat fat 4 g | Fiber 1 g | Sodium 280 mg

Lemony White Bean Bruschetta

MAKES **8 SERVINGS**

1 (8-oz.) long loaf whole wheat baguette

1 lemon

1 (15- to 19-oz.) can white kidney beans (cannellini), rinsed and drained

1 Tbsp. olive oil

¼ tsp. salt

⅛ tsp. coarsely ground pepper

1 Tbsp. plus 1 tsp. chopped fresh parsley leaves

2 cloves garlic, each cut in half

1. Prepare charcoal fire or preheat gas grill for direct grilling over medium heat.

2. Meanwhile, slice bread diagonally into ½-in.-thick slices; reserve ends for making bread crumbs another day.

3. From lemon, grate ½ tsp. peel and squeeze 1 Tbsp. juice. In medium bowl, with fork, lightly mash beans with lemon juice and peel, oil, salt, pepper, and 1 Tbsp. parsley.

4. Place bread slices on grill rack and cook 2 to 3 min. or until lightly toasted on both sides. Rub 1 side of each toast slice with cut side of garlic.

5. Just before serving, top garlic-rubbed side of toast with bean mixture and sprinkle with remaining parsley.

PER SERVING ||||||||||||||||||||||||||||||||||||||||||||||||||||||||||||||||||||||||||||||||||||
Calories 140 | Protein 5 g | Carbohydrate 23 g | Total fat 3 g
Sat fat 1 g | Fiber 3 g | Sodium 310 mg

Mediterranean Marinated Shrimp

MAKES **12 SERVINGS**

½ c. olive oil

1 Tbsp. grated lemon zest

½ c. lemon juice

1 tsp. salt

1 tsp. dried oregano

½ tsp. crushed red pepper

½ tsp. minced garlic

2 lbs. peeled and deveined shrimp (16 to 21 pieces per lb.), thawed if frozen

1 (7-oz.) jar roasted peppers, drained and sliced

¼ c. chopped parsley

½ c. crumbled feta cheese

1. Combine oil, lemon zest, lemon juice, salt, oregano, red pepper and garlic in large zip-top bag; seal bag, then turn a few times to mix. Set aside.

2. Add shrimp to large deep skillet of boiling water. Reduce heat and cook 1 to 2 min. or until just cooked through. Drain; rinse under cold water and drain again.

3. Add shrimp to bag with marinade; seal and turn to coat.

4. Refrigerate overnight, turning bag occasionally. Transfer to serving bowl; stir in roasted peppers, parsley and feta, and toss.

PER SERVING ||||||||||||||||||||||||||||||||||||||||||||||||||||||||||||||||||||||||||||||||||
Calories 140 | Protein 5 g | Carbohydrate 23 g | Total fat 3 g
Sat fat 1 g | Fiber 3 g | Sodium 310 mg

Peppery Chickpeas

YIELD **1¾ CUPS** | SERVING SIZE **¼ CUP**

1 Tbsp. extra-virgin olive oil

1 (15- to 19-oz.) can garbanzo beans (chickpeas)

½ tsp. dried Italian seasoning

⅛ tsp. ground red pepper (cayenne)

¼ tsp. salt

Cocktail picks

1. In nonstick 10-in. skillet, heat oil over medium-high heat. Meanwhile, drain and rinse beans. Transfer beans to paper towels; pat completely dry.

2. Add beans, Italian seasoning, ground red pepper and salt to skillet; cook about 7 min. or until beans brown slightly, shaking pan occasionally.

3. Transfer beans to shallow bowl. Serve with cocktail picks.

PER SERVING ||||||||||||||||||||||||||||||||||||||||||||||||||||||||||||||||||||||||||||||||||||||||||
Calories 110 | Protein 5g | Carbohydrate 14g | Total fat 4g
Sat fat 0g | Fiber 4g | Sodium 410 mg

Beverages

Forget those diet-busting double martinis and Long Island iced teas you are tempted with when going out. Entertain at home instead, and serve from this list of beverages that come in at 200 calories per serving or less.

Blood Orange Mimosa

MAKES **8 SERVINGS**

2 c. fresh blood orange juice, well chilled

1 (750-ml) bottle dry Prosecco or other dry sparkling wine, well chilled

Fresh blood orange slices, for garnish

1. Into each of 8 champagne flutes or tall juice glasses, pour ¼ c. juice. Top off each glass with some Prosecco and, if you like, attach a slice of blood orange to rim of each glass.

PER SERVING ||||||||||||||||||||||||||||||||||||||||||||||||||||||||||||||||||||||||||||||||||
Calories 100 | Protein 0 g | Carbohydrate 8 g | Total fat 0 g
Sat fat 0 g | Fiber 0 g | Sodium 0 mg

Minty Iced Tea

MAKES **8 SERVINGS**

8 tea bags, tags removed

8 sprigs fresh mint, plus additional for serving

¼ c. fresh lime juice, (2 to 3 limes)

Ice cubes

1. In covered 3-qt. saucepan, heat 4 c. cold water to boiling over high heat. Remove from heat; stir in tea bags and mint. Cover and let steep 5 min.

2. Stir tea; remove tea bags and mint. Into large pitcher with tight-fitting lid, pour tea, lime juice and 4 c. cold water. Makes 8 cups. Cover and let stand until ready to serve or overnight. (Do not refrigerate, or tea will become cloudy. If that happens, add up to 1 c. boiling water, gradually, stirring until tea clears.) Serve over ice with mint.

PER SERVING |||||||||||||||||||||||||||||||||||||||||||||||||||||||||||||||||||||||||||||||||||||||||||||||||||||||||||
Calories 0 | Protein 0 g | Carbohydrate 0 g | Total fat 0 g | Sat fat 0 g
Fiber 0 g | Sodium 10 mg

Mulled-Wine Sangria

MAKES 6 TO 8 SERVINGS

1 (750-ml) bottle red wine

2 c. cranberry juice

1 c. fresh or frozen
cranberries

½ c. orange liqueur

½ c. packed light-brown
sugar

2 cinnamon sticks

1 strip (wide) orange peel

2 green apples, chopped

1. Put wine, cranberry juice, cranberries, orange liqueur, brown sugar, cinnamon sticks and orange peel in large saucepan.

2. Bring to a simmer over medium heat and cook, stirring, 5 min., or until the sugar dissolves.

3. Remove from heat; set aside for 15 min.

4. Stir apples into mulled wine.

5. Serve immediately or refrigerate and serve chilled.

PER SERVING ||||||||||||||||||||||||||||||||||||||||||||||||||||||||||||||||||||||||||||||||

Calories 250 | Protein 0 g | Carbohydrate 38 g | Total fat 0 g
Sat fat 0 g | Fiber 2 g | Sodium 10 mg

Pomegranate Cosmo

MAKES 4 SERVINGS

1 c. vodka

1 c. pomegranate-cranberry
juice blend

¼ c. orange liqueur

3 Tbsp. fresh lime juice

Lime twists, for garnish

1. Put vodka, pomegranate juice, orange liqueur and lime juice in large liquid measuring cup or other pitcher.

2. Add ice and stir 30 sec. or until cold; strain into chilled martini glasses.

3. Garnish with lime twists.

PER SERVING ||||||||||||||||||||||||||||||||||||||||||||||||||||||||||||||||||||||||||||||||

Calories 200 | Protein 0 g | Carbohydrate 13 g | Total fat 0 g
Sat fat 0 g | Fiber 0 g | Sodium 5 mg

Pomegranate Sangria

MAKES **8 SERVINGS**

1 (750-ml) bottle semidry
   Riesling or other white wine

1 c. pomegranate juice

¼ c. orange liqueur

1 orange, cut into ¼-in. slices

1 Granny Smith apple, cored
   and thinly sliced

½ c. pomegranate seeds

Seltzer or club soda (optional)

1. In large pitcher or punch bowl, combine Riesling, pomegranate juice and orange liqueur. Add orange and apple slices, and pomegranate seeds; stir well.

2. Cover and refrigerate mixture for at least 3 hrs. or overnight.

3. Divide among glasses and top off with seltzer or club soda, if desired.

PER SERVING |||||||||||||||||||||||||||||||||||||||||||||||||||||||||||||||||||||||||||||
Calories 150 | Protein 1 g | Carbohydrate 18 g | Total fat 0 g
Sat fat 0 g | Fiber 1 g | Sodium 0 mg

Simple Sangria

MAKES **12 SERVINGS**

1 (1½-liter) bottle red wine

1½ c. fresh orange juice

⅓ c. brandy

⅓ c. sugar

2 nectarines, pitted and
   cut into wedges

1 orange, cut in half then
   sliced

1 lemon, sliced

1 Kirby (pickling)
   cucumber, sliced

3 c. seltzer or club
   soda, chilled

 Ice cubes

1. In 3- to 4-qt. pitcher, combine wine, orange juice, brandy and sugar; stir until sugar dissolves.

2. Stir in fruits and cucumber. Cover and refrigerate until well chilled, at least 3 hrs. or overnight.

3. To serve, stir seltzer into pitcher. Fill glasses with ice and pour sangria.

PER SERVING |||||||||||||||||||||||||||||||||||||||||||||||||||||||||||||||||||||||||||||
Calories 170 | Protein 1 g | Carbohydrate 15 g | Total fat 0 g
Sat fat 0 g | Fiber 1 g | Sodium 5 mg

Metric Equivalents

The recipes in this book use the standard United States method for measuring liquid and dry or solid ingredients (teaspoons, tablespoons, and cups). The information on these charts is provided to help cooks outside the U.S. successfully use these recipes. All equivalents are approximate.

Metric Equivalents for Different Types of Ingredients

A standard cup measure of a dry or solid ingredient will vary in weight depending on the type of ingredient. A standard cup of liquid is the same volume for any type of liquid. Use the following chart when converting standard cup measures to grams (weight) or milliliters (volume).

Standard Cup	Fine Powder (e.g. flour)	Grain (e.g. rice)	Granular (e.g. granulated sugar)	Liquid Solids (e.g.butter)	Liquid (e.g. milk)
1	140 g	150 g	190 g	200 g	240 ml
¾	105 g	113 g	143 g	150 g	180 ml
⅔	93 g	100 g	133 g	160 g	160 ml
½	70 g	75 g	95 g	100 g	120 ml
⅓	47 g	50 g	63 g	67 g	80 ml
¼	35 g	38 g	48 g	50 g	60 ml
⅛	18 g	19 g	24 g	25 g	30 ml

Equivalents for Liquid Ingredients by Volume

¼ tsp. =				1 ml	
½ tsp. =				2 ml	
1 tsp. =				5 ml	
3 tsp. =	1 Tbsp. =		½ fl. oz. =	15 ml	
	2 Tbsp. =	⅛ cup =	1 fl. oz. =	30 ml	
	4 Tbsp. =	¼ cup =	2 fl. oz. =	60 ml	
	5⅓ Tbsp.=	⅓ cup =	3 fl. oz. =	80 ml	
	8 Tbsp. =	½ cup =	4 fl. oz. =	120 ml	
	10⅔ Tbsp.=	⅔ cup =	5 fl. oz. =	160 ml	
	12 Tbsp. =	¾ cup =	6 fl. oz. =	180 ml	
	16 Tbsp. =	1 cup =	8 fl. oz. =	240 ml	
	1 pt. =	2 cups =	16 fl. oz. =	480 ml	
	1 qt. =	4 cups =	32 fl. oz. =	960 ml	
			33 fl. oz. =	1000 ml	1L

Equivalents for Dry Ingredients by Weight

To convert ounces to grams, multiply the number of ounces by 30.

1 oz. =	$\frac{1}{16}$ lb. =	30 g
4 oz. =	¼ lb. =	120 g
8 oz. =	½ lb. =	240 g
12 oz. =	¾ lb. =	360 g
16 oz. =	1 lb. =	480 g

Equivalents for Cooking/Oven Temperatures

	Farenheit	Celsius	Gas Mark
Freeze Water	32°F	0°C	
Room Temperature	68°F	20°C	
Boil Water	212°F	100°C	
Bake	325°F	160°C	3
	350°F	180°C	4
	375°F	190°C	5
	400°F	200°C	6
	425°F	220°C	7
	450°F	230°C	8
Broil			Grill

Index

Note: Page numbers in *italics* indicate recipes.

About the Authors

Samantha Cassetty, M.S., R.D.

Director of nutrition, Luvo; formerly nutrition director, *Good Housekeeping*
and Good Housekeeping Research Institute

Samantha served as the nutrition director of *Good Housekeeping* for six years, and as a registered dietitian, she was the perfect person to develop the meal plan that anchors this book, and she was also our go-to expert on all the latest nutrition news and facts. She knows which foods have the highest levels of vitamins and antioxidants while also being low in calories and delicious to eat— the exact combination that a Mediterranean diet is known for.

During her time at *Good Housekeeping*, Samantha's nutrition and diet expertise was behind the magazine's monthly Nutrition News and Drop 5 Lbs columns as well as all of GH's weight-loss plans—including the one in our *New York Times* best-selling *7 Years Younger: The Revolutionary 7-Week Anti-Aging Plan.* In addition, she oversaw the food category for the Good Housekeeping Seal. Samantha has also been tapped as an expert on healthy eating on a variety of local and syndicated television and radio shows and has made a number of appearances on national television programs, including *Today, Dr. Oz.,* and *CBS Sunday Morning.* Samantha's nutrition and diet expertise is also on The Cooking Channel's *Drop 5 Lbs with Good Housekeeping,* where she serves as the nutrition correspondent.

Debora Yost

Debora Yost is a veteran health journalist with 30 years of experience. During that time she has created and written or edited more than 300 healthy lifestyle books that have sold more than 30 million copies. Her latest idea is *The Girlfriends Diet.* Prior to going out on her own, Debora was vice president and editor in chief of Prevention Magazine Health Books and senior vice president and publisher of Prentice Hall Direct.

Her most recent books are *Healing Spices: How to Use 50 Everyday and Exotic Spices to Boost Health and Beat Disease* and *7 Years Younger: The Anti-Aging Breakthrough Diet.*

Good Housekeeping Research Institute

The Girlfriends Diet also benefits from the expertise of the Good Housekeeping Research Institute (GHRI), which is the product-evaluation laboratory of *Good Housekeeping* magazine, with a staff of scientists, engineers, nutritionists and researchers dedicated to evaluating and testing everything from moisturizers to bedsheets to cell phones. Also part of GHRI is the test kitchen, which creates, tastes and triple-tests (at least) the thousands of recipes appearing annually in the magazine and on goodhousekeeping.com.

The institute was founded in 1900 to improve the lives of consumers and their families through education and product evaluation. It has departments specializing in consumer electronics and engineering to test appliances like flat-screen TVs and refrigerators; health, beauty and environmental sciences for beauty and hair care products; textiles, paper and plastics, which analyzes fiber-based products like sweaters, suitcases and backpacks; and the editorial test kitchens to assess foods' nutrition claims and create low-cost, family-friendly meal solutions.

The information in this book is not meant to take the place of the advice of your doctor. Before embarking on a weight loss program, you are advised to seek your doctor's counsel to make sure that the weight loss plan you choose is right for your particular needs. Further, this book's mention of products made by various companies does not imply that those companies endorse this book.

Cover design by Jill Armus
Interior design by Tara Long

Cover image: pierre bourrier / Alamy
ISBN 978-1-936297-73-3

Cataloging-in-Publication Data available from the Library of Congress

10 9 8 7 6 5 4 3 2

Published by Hearst Editions/Hearst Magazines
300 West 57th Street
New York, NY 10019

Good Housekeeping is a registered trademark of Hearst Communications, Inc.
www.goodhousekeeping.com

Distributed to the trade by Hachette Book Group

All US and Canadian orders:
Hachette Book Group
Order Department
Three Center Plaza
Boston, MA 02108
Call toll free: 1-800-759-0190
Fax toll free: 1-800-286-9471

For information regarding discounts to corporations, organizations, non-book retailers and wholesalers; mail order catalogs; and premiums, contact:
Special Markets Department
Hachette Book Group
237 Park Avenue
New York, NY 10017
Call toll free: 1-800-222-6747
Fax toll free: 1-800-222-6902

For all international orders:
Hachette Book Group
237 Park Avenue
New York, NY 10017
Tel: 212-364-1325
Fax: 800-364-0933
international@hbgusa.com

Printed in the USA